Robert Chernin Cantor

And a Time to Live

Toward Emotional Well-Being During the Crisis of Cancer

HARPER COLOPHON BOOKS

HARPER & ROW, PUBLISHERS

NEW YORK, CAMBRIDGE, HAGERSTOWN, PHILADELPHIA, SAN FRANCISCO

LONDON, MEXICO CITY, SAO PAULO, SYDNEY

For Niki
and to the Memory of Jack Cantor

"Coming to This Place" by Lawrence Fixel. Copyright © 1978 by Lawrence Fixel.

"By the waters of the woodland . . ." by Kim Chernin. Copyright © 1978 by Kim Chernin.

Poem on page 221 is reprinted by permission of the publishers and the Trustees of Amherst College from *The Poems of Emily Dickinson,* edited by Thomas H. Johnson, Cambridge, Mass.: The Belknap Press of Harvard University Press, Copyright © 1951, 1955, by the President and Fellows of Harvard College.

Poem on page 190 from "The Road Not Taken" from *The Poetry of Robert Frost* edited by Edward Connery Lathem. Copyright 1916, © 1969 by Holt, Rinehart and Winston, Inc. Copyright 1944 by Robert Frost, reprinted by permission of Holt, Rinehart and Winston, Inc.

Extract from "The Last Day of April" copyright © 1974 by Nancy Roach. Reprinted by permission of The American Cancer Society.

A hardcover edition of this book is published by Harper & Row, Publishers.

First HARPER COLOPHON edition published 1980.

ISBN: 0-06-090746-0

84 10 9 8 7 6 5 4 3 2

Contents

Part Two: The Sphere of Personal Influence

Part Three: The Sphere of Family Influence

Part Four: The Search for Meaning

Acknowledgments

I can not conceive of having written this book without the help of many people and institutions. I am primarily in debt to the hundreds and hundreds of cancer patients and family members who shared their struggles with me and thereby deepened my understanding of the human condition. This is, essentially, their courageous story. I am grateful to the Wright Institute of Berkeley, California, for providing the rich intellectual environment in which I began to integrate my thoughts about the cancer experience; to the American Cancer Society for funding so many valuable training and service programs for cancer patients; and to the University of California Medical Center for supporting the cancer rehabilitation clinics through which I began to learn about the crisis of cancer. I am particularly grateful to Thomas A. Curtis of the University of California for permitting me the time and space to pursue my interests in the emotional aspects of cancer treatment and to Robert J. Mostovoy, who graciously assumed the greater portion of my teaching and clinical responsibilities during those years. I am also deeply appreciative of my friends and colleagues at the Family Therapy Center in San Francisco. They provided warm, continuous, thoughtful and immensely helpful support.

I want to acknowledge my gratitude to the following people who made direct and important contributions to the book: Walter E. Johnson, who offered his wise pastoral philosophy in Chapter 13; Dixie B. Shipp, who (with a little help from Holly, Nancy and

Larissa) transcribed hours and hours of tapes, conducted valuable searches of the professional literature and provided a personal enthusiasm that was a source of great encouragement; Ruth V. Halley, who carefully typed the final manuscript; Rhoda A. Weyr, who convinced me that the book could be a reality and then fought for it; Frances McCullough and her editorial assistant Patricia Fairfield, who helped polish and improve it. In addition, many people read and commented on portions of the original manuscript. I am especially grateful for the intelligent and sensitive criticism of Mildred Cantor, David L. Geisinger, Walter E. Johnson, Alan and Eva Leveton, Stephanie Mathews-Simonton, Jim Purcell, Nancy Roach, Lillian Rubin and Dennis J. Zeitlin.

And lastly, I am enormously grateful to my daughter Niki who has grown into such a lovely, bright, independent young woman and of whom I am so proud. She has brought more richness than I could describe into this, my time to live.

ABOUT THE AUTHOR

Dr. Cantor received his D.M.D. from the New Jersey College of Medicine and Dentistry and his Ph.D. in Social-Clinical Psychology from the Wright Institute of Berkeley, California. He was awarded a two-year Post-Doctoral Clinical Fellowship by the American Cancer Society to pursue his studies in cancer rehabilitation at the University of California, San Francisco.

Dr. Cantor has worked with cancer patients and their families for the past seventeen years. He has conducted over fifty workshops on the emotional aspects of cancer treatment and was the Coordinator and Co-Director of the cancer rehabilitation clinic at the University of California Medical Center for ten years. He is presently in private practice at the Family Therapy Center in San Francisco.

Introduction

Then one day it's not someone else, the name on the
report of malignancy is your own . . . you clench your
teeth and try not to hear the cataract. You had thought
it was twenty miles downstream, but it's just around the
bend.

—ALLEN WHEELIS, *The Seeker*

How do I dare ask you, my reader, to explore what is probably the
most frightening of all man's afflictions? If you, your mother, father,
son, daughter, wife, husband or any other close family member has
had or now has cancer, you might understandably feel that you know
more than you ever wanted to about this dreadful disease. Yet I do
ask, I even implore you, to look more deeply into the personal crisis
of cancer.

Each of us is unique. So too is our personal experience of cancer
and so too are our continuing aspirations. Some of us want only to
be comforted and reassured. Others yearn for more information and
for new ways of thinking about the intense emotions that accompany
diagnosis and treatment. Still others experience a frustrating impasse, are full of sadness and outrage, do not know how to go on.
I believe this book has much that is of value for those who want to
offer or receive reassurance, for those who hunger for deeper insights and for those who feel depressed, trapped and anxiously burdened.

The word *crisis* is written with two characters in Chinese. One symbol represents *danger,* the other stands for *opportunity.* [1] The diagnosis of cancer is one of the worst crises that can assault our lives. We face not only a threatening prospect of pain and death, but enter upon a forbidding path of potential loss. The dangers are distressingly apparent; the opportunities lie hidden within the stressful demands of the cancer crisis. To be *unaware* of choice and opportunity is to experience oneself as a helpless victim—one of the most unpleasant of all imaginable possibilities. And yet choice and opportunity are often disregarded and the role of victim passively selected. To be *aware* of ever-present opportunity is difficult indeed, for it requires confronting many of the painful doubts, complex choices and personal responsibilities that accompany all efforts to become the architect of one's fate. It is never easy to struggle with doubt or assume responsibility for complex decisions; such struggles are particularly difficult during the cancer crisis. But it is possible to assume responsibility for one's life even under the most trying circumstances. And it is this process of self-confrontation that leads to the creation of unexpected opportunity.

In the midst of joyful celebration, the leaders of one ancient civilization would place a skull before their guests as a reminder of man's transitory existence. [2] It was intended as a testament to human mortality; an awareness they believed would deepen, enrich and heighten the fleeting moments of life. Similarly, we can attempt to experience the diagnosis of cancer as a timely reminder that we will not live forever. The awareness of our mortality is thrust upon us and we are faced with a fundamental choice. As cancer patients and family members, we can try to forget the frightening vision and thereby attempt to regain our innocence of death. OR each of us can pause and ask: What is it I value and want most in my life? Have I neglected or lost sight of anything important? How do I want to use this, my time to live? It matters not whether the opportunities of the cancer experience involve the preservation of what is familiar or the exploration of what is new and unfolding; we must still decide whether to acknowledge or try to ignore the skull upon the banquet table. The choice we make will determine whether or not our lives become deeper and more meaningful as a result of cancer treatment and the possible threat to our existence.

I write for those who choose to understand; for those, be they patient, friend, nurse, family member or physician, who want to examine the cancer experience and come to know it better; for those who see themselves as active participants in the process of treatment and recovery. For years I have witnessed pain and distress that need not have existed, pain and distress that did not arise directly from the fact of disease but rather from the way in which patients, families, nurses and physicians went about dealing with what the cancer meant to them. Cancer and cancer treatment are dreadful burdens to endure. And yet a great deal of the most debilitating stress is secondary to the cancer itself. The degree of active influence that can be used to reduce the stress is enormous. Most of the difficult problems faced by cancer patients are usually faced by them alone. This is so not only because of the need and respect for privacy, not usually because friends, families and doctors lack concern, rarely because of intentional neglect, but rather because everyone involved is bewildered and overwhelmed by the complex questions and demands of the cancer experience.

I have two French doors leading from my study to a small balcony overlooking a garden. One door is open, the other closed. As I write I look up and watch a bee furiously buzzing against the closed door, trying to force his way through the glass. The bee presumably can see the trees and flowers outside the door; in an effort to return to them, he lunges away within the wooden boundaries of the glass pane. Finally he drops exhausted to the wooden threshold, and then, a few moments later, flies effortlessly out the open door. Many of us similarly pursue a single, self-defeating course of action during the cancer crisis—we exhaust ourselves in vain struggle, never once having paused to recognize or to create alternatives. We often feel bewildered and overwhelmed by this crisis as a direct result of our failure to recognize inherent possibilities and concrete tasks. What a different experience it would be if we, at such a moment, voluntarily refrained from our habitual behavior, risked asking some difficult questions and then reconsidered our experience, circumstance and opportunities. This book is both an appeal to enter upon such a process of reflection and a means by which it can be done.

In *And a Time to Live* I attempt to portray the cancer experience and many of its inherent choices. Several excellent books have been written on death and dying.[3] This is not another. *And a Time to Live* is a book about preserving and even improving the quality of one's life following this dramatic threat to its continuance. The emphasis will be on understanding and ameliorating the threatening experiences of cancer treatment, experiences which cancer patients and their families share in common.

I have written the narrative as though I were talking informally with a group of intelligent people unschooled in medical and psychological jargon. But it is a demanding book. I will ask you to consider deeply, to confront difficult ideas and to be honestly introspective. I will also ask you to think in terms of themes and patterns. We will explore possibilities, clarify alternatives, search for opportunities and discover new perspectives.

There are four large sections. Part One, *The Cancer Experience*, portrays the wide range of possible responses to the diagnosis and treatment of cancer. Part Two, *The Sphere of Personal Influence*, presents tasks and perspectives by which *individuals* can maintain or regain their sense of personal authority and competence. Part Three, *The Sphere of Family Influence*, discusses the impact of cancer treatment on different kinds of *marriages* and suggests ways in which this type of stress can be resolved. Part Four, *The Search for Meaning*, provides many examples of and explores several pathways toward the most life-sustaining force in existence—the evolution of personal meaning.

Most of us have not taken the time to develop a comprehensive personal philosophy of life. We therefore lack a framework within which to consider the deeper experiences and the larger questions evoked by the cancer crisis. We find it difficult to discuss these emergent, undefined but intensely important feelings with others. Being relatively unprepared, we become mute in the face of so much that is new to us. I hope that the concepts and experiences presented in this book will provide a language with which we may approach these larger issues and share them together—a language that might serve both as a bridge to others and a bridge toward the experiences themselves. My hope is that these ideas will germinate and grow and develop their unique application.

I think of *patients* who have said to me: "I feel so bewildered by the whole thing. I don't know why I'm so sad and irritable. I shouldn't be this way. I've always been able to deal with things. Now I'm afraid and confused." For them, I hope the book will provide a context to understand the cancer experience, to reflect on themselves less harshly. Once we are able to understand experience without judging it, we have taken the first step toward reestablishing emotional order and competence. And I think of patients who have said: "So what if I know more about why I'm having so much difficulty. That's not what I need at all. I want help in dealing with the problems, help to get me beyond them." I agree. It is not enough to portray helplessness. Meaningful ways to resolve the feelings of helplessness must be offered. I therefore seek to establish certain general understandings and to suggest possible resolutions for many of the emotions that make up the cancer experience. This approach is more than theoretical. The ways of proceeding beyond the cancer crisis have largely been drawn from the experiences of cancer patients and their families; they are valuable tools of understanding and means of resolution which have already proved to be effective.

I recall *family members* who have said to me: "I feel lost and unable to help. It is as if a wall has come up between us and I can't find a way to reach out." For them, I hope the book will provide an understanding of how this difficulty can arise and will offer a new perspective on those efforts which have some promise of overcoming emotional isolation. It may help for a family to read the book together—discuss the ideas, argue, agree, disagree; the shared discourse is essential.

I think of *students* in the health professions who have said to me: "I'm not a psychologist. Why do you keep telling me to evaluate each individual and respond with sensitivity to each need? I don't know how to evaluate. I haven't the skills." For them, I hope the book will provide a framework, an instructive context, a new way of approaching their patients and themselves, a guide as to realistic limits of responsibility.

I am also often asked: "Why do you consult with cancer patients and their families? It's so depressing." It is true that a great deal of stress and pain permeate the cancer experience—pain and stress which I must share. And yet it seems to me that a life force of unusual intensity is released whenever any of us is threatened by death. I have shared the moments when this life force came surging through years of inhibition and restraint, flooding everyone with awe and wonder. I have helped patients and their families look deeply into themselves, wrestle with the most profound questions affecting their lives and come to terms with their own values and ideals. I have learned and grown with them. Far from being depressing, I have experienced these moments of intense feeling and profound confrontation as rich and inspiring. To me, they are among the finest experiences of our humanity. I hope, above all else, that some of this affirmation is conveyed in the book you are about to read.

PART ONE

The Cancer Experience

The emotional experiences associated with cancer and cancer treatment are so painful and frightening that you may well recoil from reading this first portion of the book. There is a great deal of reassuring information in the sections that follow. But it is only by examining our *responses* to cancer that we shall be able to attain authentic reassurance about our ability to survive with a renewed sense of personal competence. When we understand these experiences we can search for answers to the strange fact that cancer frightens and horrifies us much more than other diseases which are both more prevalent and more lethal. Only then can we look at the origins of depression and at its hidden relationship to anger. Only then can we come to know the healing process of grief and thereby separate it from the passive resignation of depression. These portraits of the cancer experience will also expose many hidden fears which derive disruptive power solely from our lack of awareness. Let us therefore examine these experiences together and evolve an understanding that will provide a foundation upon which personal authority, competence, influence and meaning can be developed and enlarged.

1

The Dark Cloud of Unknowing

She shook for terror and her fear of the unknown sur-
passed by far, the fear of any peril that ever she con-
ceived.

—ERICH NEUMANN, *Amor and the Psyche*

The Virulent Image

It is quite evident that cancer is one of the major life-threatening
diseases that afflict mankind. As with any other threat to life and
well-being, those afflicted come to know a variety of vivid and frightening experiences. These stressful responses are consistent whether
the diagnosis be cancer, heart disease, diabetes or any other life-
threatening illness. But there are important differences of degree.
We are all aware that the diagnosis of cancer, just the image of
cancer, touches and frightens us more than the others. Why is this
so?

Heart disease and stroke account for nearly 50 percent of all
deaths in the United States. Cancer accounts for less than 17 percent.[1] Certainly we are concerned about heart disease and stroke,
worried about these diseases of the circulatory system that are so
pervasive and so debilitating, that kill nearly one of every two of us.
But we are terrified of cancer, not heart disease. A recent survey
showed that Californians are more afraid of cancer than of any single
danger in the world, including violent crimes and atomic war.[2] The

word *cancer* strikes terror into every adult for we share a similar image; a vision not only of a fatal disease, but of a devouring, relentless force, a force beyond our ability to control, a force that threatens to carry us into the terrifying unknown.

What is it about cancer that evokes this dreadful vision? I believe the answers have to do with issues of control, with specific sources of anxiety and with a disowned aspect in each of us that Jung calls the "shadow." The diagnosis of cancer more than that of any other disease can strip away our sense of control and release an assault of frightening possibilities, some known, some unknown, but all seemingly beyond our sphere of influence. There are many potential responses. These various attitudes fall into categories reminiscent of the fable of the twins who are about to be born. One says, "I don't want to go anywhere. I can't imagine what's out there. It is scary and *I don't want to find out."* The other twin replies, "Maybe, but I am *more curious than frightened,* so here I go."

The twins, like all of us, really have no choice; ready or not, with fear, curiosity or both, we are expelled from the womb's warm safety, forced to enter a new world of experience. As of now, we cannot choose to remain unborn, never to age, never to die. And we cannot elect never to get cancer or experience its multiple consequences. But we can decide whether to go about our lives like the first twin or the second. We can choose the attitudes we will assume during the cancer crisis and thereby influence what kind of experience it will be.

Cancer and Loss of Control

The Benefits of Clarity and Effectiveness. Most of us need to experience some sense of control over our destinies. We need to feel that what we do and say will have substantial effect on the events of our lives. We need to make sense of ourselves and our surroundings. We therefore try to anticipate what will happen to us; we infer cause and effect and explain the events that befall us. Competence and personal authority issue from these efforts of understanding and mastery. They are not idle games that we play at our leisure. They are among the inherent tasks of human existence. Unless each of us feels some potency, some ability to understand and have effect, we experience ourselves as the passive victims of outside forces, we know ourselves to be without significance.

The diagnosis of cancer is usually experienced as just such a devastating blow to our feelings of control and effectiveness. In this respect, it is experienced quite differently from other diseases which do not seem so impervious to personal influence. And, in addition, as long as cancer remains an unknown force, it can easily become a screen onto which our worst fears and fantasies are projected.

The False Equation. The basic assumption that cancer is equivalent with death contributes to the experience of diminishing control. In 1974, approximately 218,000 Americans were cured of cancer while 355,000 died of it.[3] At this time, there were already 1,500,000 American cancer patients who had been successfully treated. Cancer is a major life-threatening disease; it most certainly kills people. But most of our assumptions grossly exaggerate its impact. In a recent Gallup poll,[4] only 8 percent of the women questioned came reasonably close to guessing the correct incidence of breast cancer. The great majority thought the chances of getting it were two to three times what they really are. Most of us simply equate the diagnosis of cancer with death. Since the statistics do not support this equation, the assumption must be the product of our selective interpretation.

Assumptions based on subtle interpretation of "facts" are common. Two newspapers report the same incident: A small submarine with four scientists aboard is trapped on the ocean floor off Florida. The San Francisco *Examiner* headline reads: "Two Found Dead of Cold in Midget Submarine." On the same day a San Francisco *Chronicle* headline reads: "Tiny Sub Rescued—Two Crewmen Safe."[5] These unintentional interpretations are remarkably different. Those who read the *Examiner* got an overall impression of death; those who read the *Chronicle* one of rescue and survival.

Most of us have known someone who died of cancer. The death remains vivid and confirms our worst fears. But the survivors, those who have been treated and cured of cancer, are usually overlooked. The assumption that cancer kills almost everyone takes hold and haunts us. But we are, in part, responsible for creating this image by means of our selective awareness.

Assumptions about treatment contribute to the same image. It is possible to sense one's active influence on the clinical course of heart disease, stroke or diabetes. Medication, diet, physical therapy and exercise all have effect on these illnesses. But the image of cancer affords no such sense of active influence and the assumption is made that cancer is a force beyond one's control, a force that cannot be altered by physical or emotional activities. This assumption gives rise to debilitating anxiety and despair. In many respects it is also incorrect, and in a later chapter we will examine some of the ways in which an active influence can be asserted.

Fair Game for the Guardians. Another source contributing to the experience of diminishing control has to do with hospitalization, with the loss of familiar things and conventional restraints. The surgical ward of a hospital has been correctly likened to a "displaced persons camp." The diagnosis of cancer simply intensifies the experience. Any of us entering such a ward find ourselves without normal social guidelines. Nurses and physicians expose, examine, squeeze, probe and manipulate any part of us they choose to. Suddenly what always seemed appropriate is no longer valid and we must ask ourselves to accept behavior that would normally be a terrible affront to our sense of integrity. Our understanding of what is appropriate to a surgical ward does not always dispel this sense of violation. Many levels of the experience are evoked by the images of Lawrence Fixel's poem "Coming to This Place."[6]

> Arriving first as visitors
> where white uniforms confirm
> the gleam of corridors   the filtered air
> We follow the formal logic
> that charts the iron bed: time of departure

date of return   to the "normal & the sane"
To suddenly find ourselves—no longer observers—
fair game for the guardians: being prepared
for the strict regime of pills & needles
fitted for the robe   that needs no laundering. . . .

Unwilling unready to give up
the random identity of street clothes
we protest: this single-minded realm
leaves nothing for the special grace of being—
But find the schedule timed
for the convenience   of those whose skill
with serving spoon & knife   validates the course
of treatment—however long it takes.

Coming to this place   reserved for us
by pure rotation: confined under the light
that leaves no room   to wander in
we watch the gestures   of ritualized actors
who perform as if   there is no breathing space
                                   beyond the shadows

Hospitalization is a "single-minded realm" that leaves "nothing
for the special grace of being." Identity and uniqueness are reduced
to biological anomalies, and the dramatic loss of one's identity can
be extremely painful to experience.

At times the distress of hospitalization is greater for the onlooker,
as we may see from this example: "[Mama] had an open hospital
nightdress and she did not mind that her wrinkled belly, crisscrossed
with tiny lines and her bald pubis showed. 'I no longer have any sort
of shame' she observed in a surprised voice. 'You are perfectly right
not to have any' I said. But I turned away . . . the sight of my
mother's nakedness had jarred me. . . . I was astonished at the
violence of my distress."[7] In this instance, no sense of loss or violation was felt by the patient. But her daughter was forced to suffer
a vision of her mother "reduced by her capitulation to being a body
and nothing more."

Derivatives of Distance. I have often heard the wives and husbands of cancer patients describe feelings of losing control. The

diagnosis and outcome of treatment have enormous importance for them. That the tumor is located in a loved one can be experienced with ambivalence. Family members often wish that they had the cancer themselves. One husband said: "This terrible thing has come into my life and it's as if I can't get at it. Margaret is so different from me and she won't do the things I'm convinced would help. I can't do anything about the cancer but nag her and that just makes her angrier and things get worse."[8]* The wish to take on the suffering himself and the need to make her do what he wants are both, in part, efforts at recapturing some sense of being in control. Many parents would also gladly accept their child's disease; many children wish to save their parents when they are so afflicted. In addition to these genuine offerings of love and sacrifice, there is the same hidden hope that control might be reestablished and the sense of chaos might thereby be less difficult to deal with.

Forms of the Unexpected. A loss of control often results from the experience of unexpected events. Surgeons can neglect to prepare a patient properly; patients can "tune out" what they don't want to hear. The shock of discovering the extent of surgery can trigger great resentment and the feeling of not having had sufficient control over one's life. "I wouldn't have let him operate if I knew he would take so much of me. I would rather have died."[9] "I kind of expected to lose my breast, but I didn't think they would cut so high. That's what really disturbs me. It's so horrible and it shows, everyone can see."[10] Knowing what to expect provides stability and a sense of control. Unexpected shocks disrupt this sense of control.

Many people are able to prepare themselves for what takes place during hospitalization. Patients feel exhausted and numb while in the hospital. Their families visit, bring flowers, encourage them; all

*The illustrations and quotes that I use throughout the book come from workshops and therapy hours with cancer patients and their families, from seminars with health professionals working with cancer patients, from my own experiences and from examples cited in the literature. I have changed all identifying details, including, at times, the age and even the sex of the people involved. However, I have not changed the words themselves, nor have I changed any details that would alter their meaning in context.

accept temporary hospitalization. There is a comforting hope that the return home will bring back a time with "things as they used to be." They are therefore unprepared for what can happen following discharge. As one woman said: "Anybody who's in the hospital is sick with something. You have plenty of company and it makes a difference. You don't think about it until you get home."[11] The full emotional impact often waits until a patient is home, safe, surrounded by the familiar and feeling more in control. It is then that the fears and fantasies and dreaded consequences are permitted to come pouring into awareness. Even the physical realities are often first acknowledged at home. "The thought goes through your mind, are you going to stay together? The pull is that terrific."[12] or "When I got home I found I couldn't even sit up without aid. I had never noticed that in the hospital."[13] Inner conflicts can emerge: "There I was at home in bed, just a terrible burden to everyone. But at the same time I resented them for going on with their lives. I didn't want them to bother, I really wanted to be alone most of the time anyway, but I still wanted them to take care of me. Isn't that crazy?"[14] No, it is not crazy at all; but these apparently contradictory feelings are often unexpected and therefore they can be extremely unnerving.

Once healing and recovery have been completed there are other unexpected situations that trigger a sense of having lost control. When a disfigurement is visible, negative reactions can be anticipated and strategies to deal with these public responses can be developed. But most cancer patients are not visibly disfigured. Their treatment and permanent surgical wounds are hidden. They are therefore secretly "discreditable"[15] and must face the difficult questions of whether and who and when to tell about their treatment. They may not meet prejudice directly. But they are afraid that people who know and accept them might be repelled should they find out that they have had cancer. "Since my colostomy I've become like a detective. I watch for any sign of suspiciousness. Do they know? Can they hear or smell me? Are they making believe they don't know? Would they care if they did know? The most damnable thing is I never know what to expect and there's nothing I can do about it. I don't seem to be able to relax anywhere but home."[16] A woman who had a mastectomy said: "I've just started seeing some-one. Do I announce I'm missing a breast? I'm afraid he'll discover it before I tell him. But why should I have to tell him before I even know if I really care for him and want to sleep with him?"[17] A man looking for employment said: "I'm convinced that if they know I've had cancer they'll never hire me. And yet I don't want to start off on a lie."[18]

A great deal of the distress surrounding these issues of disclosure arises from the fact that we are unable to anticipate how people will feel and how they might react. In such circumstances, some former cancer patients become belligerent, prepare for the worst and wait vigilantly. Others hope for the best, strive to accept their vulnerability and to ignore all but the most intrusive responses. But anyone who finds himself in these unexpected circumstances will understandably begin to experience a lessening of control over his life.

Evocation of the Irrational. Cancer seems irrational and evokes the irrational. It is closely related to the unknown, to the dark, unfathomable experiences of man. It is particularly confusing in the context of our highly rational culture. Even when cancer-causing agents such as nicotine, radiation or alcohol are present, there is still a mysterious random selection of exposed individuals. There is so much about cancer that does not make sense, so much that leaps out of control. On learning that her mother had untreatable cancer, Simone de Beauvoir wrote: "I had understood all my sorrows up until that night: even when they flowed over my head, I recognized myself in them. This time my despair escaped from my control: someone other than myself was weeping in me. I talked to Sartre about my mother's mouth as I had seen it that morning . . . and he told me that my own mouth was not obeying me any more: I had put Maman's mouth on my face and in spite of myself I copied its movements."[19]

This mood and experience are not uncommon. To be "possessed" by such feelings is temporarily to surrender conscious control for the purpose of serving a greater emotional need. Such surrender may be difficult and terrifying. The mother of a leukemic child said: "I really wanted to cry out but I couldn't verbalize it and I was afraid I'd lose control. The hardest part is carrying it around for so long."[20] This woman never found out what "it" was because the conflict between controlling her feelings and expressing them was too intense. Other mothers are more open to the irrational. One mother of a leukemic child said to me: "Every mother that I talked to 'knew' long before the diagnosis was made that something was wrong. One didn't send out birth announcements, another hovered over her child, others felt months before the diagnosis that their child had leukemia. I myself had this experience. I felt it and I knew it and I was prepared. Even before Martin was born I felt I was to be faced with a greater challenge than caring for a new baby. Most of these mothers, including me, would never dare tell their doctor, but they all admit these feelings to each other."[21] We will never know for sure just how "true" such claims might be, how many fears and premonitions exactly like these go unfulfilled. But, faced with so little control, with so much "not knowing," the irrational areas of our experience, paradoxically, can offer comfort. The mothers described above temporarily traded their familiar logic for a different kind of nonrational knowledge that brought them some measure of control.

Cancer can and usually does evoke the irrational. It is frightening to feel out of control, but denial of one's experience or blind adherence to some ideal of rationality can intensify fearful fantasies and result in a yet more incapacitating sense of being out of control. There is no "normal" way to react to the cancer experience. Our nonrational experiences also have some purpose which we must try to accept and understand. But for certain people any intense experience seems irrational. These are individuals who live lives devoid of strong emotion, lives in which potential highs and lows are minimized and a comfortable midrange of feeling is achieved. Such people are strangers to intense emotion, be it great joy or sorrow. However, the cancer experience can destroy the most carefully arranged lives and create an inner tidal wave of feelings. The anguish of sudden or potential loss, the jarring realization of what is deeply valued, a rush of illuminated love—all can be both frightening and extremely difficult to experience. Intense and unfamiliar emotions of this kind can give rise to great anxiety. In these instances, the grief or love is not at all irrational; it is only unexpected, unfamiliar and therefore frightening.

However, the inability to know "for sure" when or if the cancer will reappear is probably the most powerful "disrupter" of all. A patient free from any evidence of cancer describes it as his Sword of Damocles. "I just can't live my life as before. The idea that it might come back hangs over my head all the time. No matter what I do, I can't seem to get out from under it."[22] A patient about to begin chemotherapy after his third remission refers to another Greek myth and says he feels like Sisyphus: "Here I go again, back down at the bottom of the mountain starting all over . . . each time feeling a little weaker, but pushing my way up again."[23] This experience of never knowing "for sure" gives rise to a sense that one has received an "indeterminate sentence." It is not unlike the sensation reported by certain prisoners who feel as if a line had been drawn through their previous life, as if everything of value had been taken away. In such a state, prisoners often put on "emotional armor," concentrate on sheer self-preservation and remain tormented by feelings of inferiority.[24] The fear of recurrence in cancer patients and their families can produce similar feelings, and it can be difficult to reestablish a sense of control over one's life in the midst of this experience of having received an "indeterminate sentence" of good health. The sense of losing control produces considerable anxiety. And yet it is far from being the only source of anxiety during the siege of cancer.

Cancer and Anxiety

The Force of Fantasy. The diagnosis of cancer carries a known force into our lives, a force that frightens all of us. In addition, fantasies flood into an uncertain void and the anticipation of these imagined events can produce more anxiety than the realities of diagnosis and ensuing treatment.

For primitive man, living in a world of physical danger, anxiety was a much-needed asset; the alarm response of "fight or flight" had survival value for him. In our society, the anxiety response often serves no useful purpose. A recent study showed that half of all the prescriptions written in the United States were not for specific diseases. They were for drugs that reduced anxiety.[25] Far from being a survival response, anxiety has become a modern plague. What is true for modern life generally is true for the cancer experience specifically. The excessive anxiety evoked by the image of cancer can be, at times, more stressful and more damaging to the quality of one's life than the disease itself.

The simple, physical example of a splinter illustrates this point quite well. If a dirty sliver of wood penetrates the skin, the tissue around it will become inflamed. If it is not removed, a boil can develop. This healthy barricade is adaptive, for it prevents any further spread of infection or infiltration of toxins that might possibly be carried by the splinter. But at times the body reactions are disproportionate to the assault. When this happens, the excessive inflammation, not the splinter, becomes the main cause of what we experience as disease. In fact, the endocrine response to the originally innocuous splinter can become so intense as to cause damage to organs in distant parts of the body.[26] This type of physical overreaction has its emotional counterpart. The anxiety evoked by the diagnosis of cancer can become the primary experience of the disease. When this happens, anxiety has not prepared us for action; it has produced an apprehensive self-absorption that obscures the very nature of what threatens us.

Fear, Anxiety and the Image of Cancer. Fear is usually regarded as a reaction to objective danger: a car swerves out of control, a malignant growth is detected. *Anxiety* is more typically regarded as a reaction to imagined danger: what if the brakes of the car fail, what if the cancer is untreatable, what if the surgery makes me unworthy of love and respect? However, the distinction between fear and anxiety becomes meaningless in terms of felt experience. To be in the grip of severe anxiety is to experience one of the most unpleasant and distressful emotional states known to man. One can feel great turmoil and agitation, a racing heart, sweaty palms, a need for frequent urination, waves of self-doubt and an inability to rest or relax. Regardless of the source of the danger, be it "real" or "imaginary," the emotion of severe anxiety can be terrifying, and not knowing the source of it can be the most terrifying experience of all. Many of us therefore paradoxically find specific fantasies easier to bear than the specter of the unknown. These concrete images tend to reduce the extreme anxiety and terror of what seems "unknowable." But they can cause, like the boil as a response to the innocuous splinter, more distress than the unknowable event and in this way become as misguided a response. The image of cancer invariably triggers a variety of anxieties only a few of which issue directly from the diagnosis and treatment of cancer. And since these anxieties have been known to cause more harm than the treated cancer, they deserve to be thoroughly investigated.

It is possible to prevent emotional debilitation and to help along the difficult process of acceptance and integration by becoming more familiar with some of these sources of anxiety and thereby minimizing their intensity. The sources to be considered include images of death, cancer treatment and abandonment. We will deal with the *management* of anxiety later. For now, let us scrutinize the sources themselves in order to make them accessible and familiar.

The Inferential Face of Death. We have already discussed the false equation of cancer and death. But, true or false, the assumptions that accompany the diagnosis of cancer inevitably place the anatomy of death before us. It is an unfamiliar presence. For most of us, the possibility of our own death or the death of a loved one has always been pushed aside or, if considered at all, has been placed in the far distant future. Even those of us who work with illness try to banish the fact of death. "In six years of nursing, I'd managed to avoid being with someone when they died. Amazing as it seems, it always happened on someone else's shift. My son was the first person I ever saw dying, and after all those experiences of just missing death, I was so unprepared. . . . I had no place to go, no way to look aside, no escape."[27]

What is so striking about the image of the resurrection of Christ is that he appeared to his disciples in his own recognizable human form and then went on to a life beyond the grave. This image represents the fulfillment of man's deepest desire not to die, and, when that must inevitably happen, to be reborn in the same form and with the same personal appearance, awareness and identity. One dreadful image of death is given by this fear of an irreversible finality to our personal form of existence.

Another image of death concerns time; our lives run out like sand passing through an hourglass. This image, which often appears following the diagnosis of cancer, can cause severe anxiety. Many of us have a lifelong sense of urgency. We live the adage "time's a-wasting, don't delay." Gray hairs, shortness of breath, wrinkles, aches and pains or the death of a family member are all warnings that time is passing. A cancer patient in his late fifties said: "I always imagined I'd do something great. I'm sure I have it in me. I think of Winston Churchill coming back from defeat to become a great statesman or Grandma Moses in her eighties becoming a great painter. But now I might not have the time. I feel like it's all gone. I am who I am, no more and no less. I will accomplish no more than what I've already done."[28] A woman in her thirties said: "I have this strong sense of being unfinished. I feel this hunger that is still unfulfilled. My time is running out and I'm afraid the cancer will take away my ability to finish something to gratify this yearning, to achieve something of value."[29]

The anxiety derived from the image of time running out is firmly attached to the idea of time as a linear and objective phenomenon. But time is a subjective, not a linear experience, as was well expressed by thirty-year-old auto-racing champion Jimmy Caruthers. While undergoing cobalt treatment for cancer, he said: "I've done more living at my age than most people who live to be a hundred."[30]

The sense of time running out has been described by many cancer patients as a central source of anxiety. Yet their anxiety could be only temporarily relieved if an extended "unit" of time were guaranteed. The experience of fulfillment clearly does not depend on large quantities of time but rather on how time is spent. As long as our personal illusion of an indefinite life span survives, we tend to dream our way into the future and ignore the reality of the present in which we might achieve our aspirations. When the image of death appears, this illusion is stripped away, the future shrinks to the reality of the present and we experience what we always feared might be true— that our lives are precisely what we are living. And so they are. But we can still choose to make them what we want them to be.

The Assault of Medical Intervention. A great many patients fear cancer treatment as much as or more than death itself; they are afraid of disfigurement, loss of social standing and pain. In many cases the treatment of cancer is more dramatic to a human being than the disease itself.[31] Add to this dramatic reality the catastrophic fantasies that infiltrate the images of treatment and it is easy to understand why so much anxiety is aroused. A hospital is sometimes envisioned as a place of healing. But more often it is thought of as a place of suffering and death. That the life-saving treatment for cancer is often more feared than the disease itself is well demonstrated by the fact that, although four out of five women know about breast self-examination and its benefits in terms of early detection and cure, only one woman in five performs this easy examination once a year.[32] The possibility that they may discover tumors is more frightening to them than the possibility of not discovering them and dying.

Until quite recently, successful cancer treatment was rarely discussed in great detail. Cultural stigma and personal modesty usually persuaded most cancer patients to hide the details of their treatment. In fact, successful cancer patients who continued active lives rarely permitted others to know that they had been treated for cancer. The candid disclosures of Mrs. Ford, Mrs. Rockefeller, Senators Humphrey and Church are a recent development. On the other hand, relatives or friends of dying cancer patients feel little inhibition and in an effort to unburden themselves often dramatically describe every detail of their relatives' illness. Our vicarious experience of cancer is usually frightening. Many of us have directly shared the difficult postoperative stress or the death of a relative (or friend) and we thereby assume a similar fate for ourselves. Prior experiences of this kind can produce graphic images of treatment, especially the pain and futility of therapy, and in doing so, add an immense burden of extra anxiety to the treatment itself. But there are often large errors in the equations we make, distorted conclusions drawn from the anxiety evoked by the image of cancer treatment. Many cured cancer patients report being surprised when their ominous prophecies go unfulfilled. "Here I am and I still can't believe it. It's so different than I imagined. My husband hardly notices, my tennis game is almost back to normal, the pain is gone. To think I almost didn't let them operate."[33]

Surgery is the most frightening of all treatment modalities. Consciously or unconsciously, everyone reacts to the recommendation of major surgery with great alarm. As the time approaches, some of us may not be able to sleep, may feel our hearts racing, suffer severe headaches, sweating attacks, diarrhea or vomiting. At other times we appear calm, but dream images reveal our fears: a city being bombed, a sewer stuffed with putrid waste, a bull being slaughtered. "I dreamt that I saw a row of what I thought were breasts. They were all distorted. I thought I was in a butcher shop and they were hung up on hooks like meat all around me."[34] Surgery and mutilation are fused, bound together in the image of a helpless victim subjected to violent assault.

All of us experience alarm at the thought of having our bodies, our physical integrity, so violated. There is understandable cause for alarm. Even though the surgical treatment is performed to save one's life, the loss of a body part constitutes a major personal loss. We want to live *and* to live intact. A part of the alarm derives from an adult's "realistic" fear, a part from a child's "irrational" one. On this more basic level, a child voice in each of us screams out a simple terror: "They're going to do something bad to me." The prospect of surgery can touch this childlike nightmare.

There are other areas of conflict and stress as well.

As long as a disease is "treatable," there is a clearly recognizable treatment goal—the elimination of the tumor, recovery and survival. Patients, their families and their physicians concur. But all of us must die someday and, therefore, all of us must reach a point when recovery and survival are not possible. The treatment goals should then become the promotion of comfort and disengagement. The difficult task of this time becomes the acceptance of approaching death. However, the point at which treatment goals change from survival to the promotion of a comfortable death is very vague indeed. Endless and distressful conflicts arise when this shift is advocated by some and opposed by others. It is easy to say that one should help a loved one accept his death, but it is extremely difficult to recognize and agree that the time has come to begin letting go. Some of the most poignant and stressful conflicts related to cancer treatment issue from the struggle between those valiantly holding on and those trying to let go. Each person perceives the circumstances differently, sometimes even self-righteously, and acts according to his perceptions. The result can be tense interpersonal warfare and growing anxiety.

The conflict can exist amidst the best of intentions, as we can see in this account by a hospital chaplain:

I remember this old white-haired patient. He was dying of cancer, and even though he was very guarded, his wife was always desperate to have me talk with him. Sven had had a lot of experience with ministers in Denmark who were life denying and very negative. But because of his wife's insistence, he would tolerate me from time to time. She was always present, always giving encouragement. I'd go by the room and I'd hear her saying: "Eat, Sven, eat; sit up and try to drink. . . ." She would not give up, even when he dropped into a deep coma. One day I was making my rounds. She wasn't there and I had turned to leave the room when he said: "Why won't she let me die?" I was really startled. I had no idea that he could speak. I asked him what he meant. "She's pushing and pushing me. Don't she know I have to die someday? I'm so tired of all this pushing," he said. I found Sven's wife in the cafeteria and joined her. I began by saying: "You know, I just had a good talk with Sven." She just about became hysterical. "You talked with him? What did he say? What did he do?" I told her that he began by saying: "Why won't she let me die?" You can imagine how upset she became. She talked about how it was her job to make him want to live. I tried to explain how much he wanted her permission to die in peace and I asked her if it were at all possible to see this as also part of her job. I was called away but saw her that evening. She said: "We had a good talk, Sven and me, about important things. I've been spending the time talking about eating when we could talk about our lives together." He maintained consciousness for several days; there was no pushing and pulling, they just spent some good time together saying their good-byes and then he once again slipped into a coma and then he died.[35]

Conflict of this nature can also exist within a parent. One anxious mother of a leukemic child said:

> My daughter is now ten, we've kept her alive for seven years, but I live in fear that one day she will say to me, "Why didn't you let me die as a baby? Now I've got to face my death." I couldn't bear it if she ever said that to me. At first I was afraid she'd die but then I became afraid she'd live beyond her innocence, afraid she would grow older and have to knowingly face dying, which is so much worse.[36]

All of us want to live and want those we love to live with us. The anxiety aroused by the conflict of wanting to hold on and wanting to let go can haunt us for many years.

As we have seen, anxiety can be triggered by the loss of control, by images of death and cancer treatment and by a variety of internal and external conflicts. These areas are all charged with strong emotion. And yet the most widespread and pervasive source of anxiety reported by cancer patients concerns another fear: abandonment.

Universal Image of Abandonment. We all make assumptions about why it is that others love and respect us. We are often convinced that certain personal attributes are responsible for whatever measure of esteem we enjoy. One says to oneself, I might be rejected if it were not for my strength, beauty, enthusiasm, dependability, sexiness, helpfulness or income. The fantasy of a lonely, barren future can become quite vivid when these attributes are threatened. The images of cancer are catastrophic as are the images of cancer treatment. The imagined catastrophic events threaten such personal attributes more than any other disease. Studies have shown that the corresponding fears of unacceptability, rejection and isolation cause greater anxiety and depression in cancer patients than do their fears of disease recurrence, pain and death.[37]

Many people feel vulnerable when their *ability to take care of others* becomes threatened. "Who will take care of my family? I can't be sick, there is no one else to take care of them. Even if the operation gets it all out, I've got to be strong and healthy. [*How do you think they will feel about taking care of you?*]* My wife won't like it at all! She's always had lots of ailments, always said, 'Thank God you're strong as an ox.' Now she won't know what to do. [*What do you imagine will happen?*] She'll try to find someone else to lean on."[38] This fantasy of abandonment proceeds from the assumption that the ability to provide security for his wife and family is what inspires their love and devotion. The assumption turned out to be false. The patient's wife, after an initial adjustment, welcomed the opportunity to assert herself and to practice her unused strengths and abilities. This man passed through an apprehensive and confusing period of time before he began to believe that his wife might continue to love and esteem him although he was an inactive recuperating cancer patient.

Many people center their fears of rejection around *lessened physical and sexual attractiveness*. One woman anticipating breast surgery said: "I feel it's disgusting in a sense. It seems like you are sexless. That's why I worry about his reaction. I feel it would be one of disgust."[39] Another about to have a hysterectomy said: "Married relations are all we've got. If I'm no good for that he'll leave me."[40] A man worried about possible post-operative loss of sexual capacity said: "And I'll be having to pimp for my wife."[41] It is an extremely rare occurrence for a man and a woman to separate because of surgically induced sexual incompatibility. But it is common for patients to have vivid fantasies of this happening. Some cancer patients fear being rejected by their children because of surgical disfigurement: "They might take a morbid interest. You know kids are sadists. They don't mean to be . . . but they are very sadistic."[42] Others fear becoming social outcasts: "The neighbors will gossip and everyone will feel sorry for me."[43] These fears can cause immeasurable distress; in general, most suicide notes describe just these feelings of loneliness and rejection. The images of cancer and cancer treatment evoke the terrible anxiety associated with these same fears.

*My questions are presented in italics throughout the book.

Unfortunately cancer patients and their families often do feel isolated. If a Mr. Smith is hospitalized following a heart attack, his family and friends will usually rally to his support, his boss will probably keep his job open if the work is not too strenuous, and the community in which he lives will most likely regard him with sympathy and interest. However, if a Mr. Jones undergoes surgery for cancer, family and friends are a little afraid to visit, confused about what they might say, and some are even concerned that he might be contagious. They are often more frightened than sympathetic. One patient expressed it succinctly: "No one wanted to hear how I felt. They couldn't handle it. They'd say, 'How are you?' as they left the room."[44]

Other forms of rejection can occur once patients return to their normal activities. A fourteen-year-old girl who had experienced a long remission had to have additional chemotherapy and then went back to school. She described her feelings and impressions in a journal:

> The first thoughts that come to mind are those of a terrifying whirlwind. I was like delicate glass to many and very few knew I was a human being trying to make the best of all happenings. . . . Huddled whispers and strange looks were beginning to catch my attention . . . it brought memories of how I was treated when I was in first grade [and] I didn't think people would be the same way when I reached thirteen or fourteen, but they were and they had a cruder way of approaching it. Some, who could not understand exactly what was going on, would say things like "that bitch has a wig, let's go pull it off." . . . All I wanted was acceptance. Was that too much to ask? Just to be treated like everyone else. It seemed at that time that in order for this to happen, Moses would have to go through the act of opening the Red Sea again. . . . I was surprised that people at school had a terrible sorrow and hope for someone who had broken an arm or fell off a ski lift or whatever else. But to encounter themselves with death or to put in perspective someone who is sentenced to die—that was too much. These hopes and feelings didn't show. It seemed that they were too frightened to even let me know that they knew what was going on.[45]

Rejection is also experienced by the families of cancer patients. "We learned about isolation. I began to understand how a minority family might feel in a WASP neighborhood. We live in a small town and news of Tommy's illness spread quickly. It became uncomfortable for us even to shop in the local market. Shoppers and clerks we had known for years suddenly became very occupied when they saw us coming."[46]

Some people are aware of their own participation in bringing about the isolation. "I wanted to talk but I didn't. If people really cared I'd just dissolve, so I pushed them away."[47] "I told Mom not to come. I was too busy keeping my act together and I was afraid I wouldn't be able to do it in front of her."[48] "I didn't believe anyone could understand so I pushed them away and then I blamed them for staying away."[49]

Imposed Dependence. A great deal of the anxiety evoked by the fear of abandonment has to do with a person's attitude toward being dependent on others. When people are told that they have cancer, they are asked, directly or by implication, to turn themselves over to the experts for treatment, to depend on them. And, following cancer treatment, there is usually a period of imposed dependence. It is a time in which all of us really do require the assistance and support of others. But these circumstances diminish our sense of independence.

There are people who take pride in being self-reliant; independent men and women whose confidence and self-esteem derive largely from being able to say to themselves: "I ask for no special favors; if need be, I can make it on my own." Such individuals are especially threatened by the dependency which cancer sometimes imposes. The sudden need to depend on another undermines the very foundations of their personal identity. This is particularly true of men in our culture, as women are permitted to feel dependent with much less shame and embarrassment. But many women also suffer the same fears, for they typically take care of others and have difficulty accepting help from their husbands and children. This was dramatically shown in one study in which recuperating mothers reported anxiety when their daughters took care of them. They felt that their temporary dependence signified old age and its attendant loneliness.[50]

On the other hand, there are people who are not at all afraid of being dependent on others. In fact, they secretly long to have someone become responsible for them. For such individuals, the diagnosis of cancer presents an opportunity to justify passivity. They insist that having cancer makes them helpless and others must therefore assume the responsibility for their care. This appeal places suffering in the service of one's need to be loved and cared for as a small, dependent child. Many of us have experienced these longings and are tempted to take advantage of situations in which we feel like injured children. When one is faced with the stress of cancer, it is often healthy and even desirable to retreat into such a protected environment. But abdicating too much responsibility for one's welfare often creates anxiety and the fear of being abandoned. The belief that we are incapable of depending on ourselves leads to predictable consequences: we fear abandonment and anxiously watch for any sign of rejection. The seeds of this kind of anxiety lie dormant in the circumstances of achieved passivity.

None of us are completely independent or completely dependent. We all experience both tendencies and have the capacity to be more or less responsible for ourselves. The cancer experience can intensify both the need for dependence and the need for independence. Great confusion results when these conflicting needs are experienced and expressed. One moment a patient might be outraged at not having been consulted and the next moment quite easily say: "You take care of things." The conflict is an unavoidable part of the cancer experience. Anxiety arises when it becomes infused by a predominating fear of being abandoned.

Cancer and the Shadow-Side

The Ominous Mask. Having examined the major potential sources of anxiety associated with cancer and cancer treatment, we still have not accounted for that extra measure of dread. There still seems to be too much fear in the image of cancer that is inexplicable. Every illness has an underlying symbolic meaning that is capable

of changing a person's image of himself. What does cancer symbol-
ize to us? What does it represent? In exploring a possible answer to
this question, I hope to account for the additional intense dread that
most of us associate with cancer. These ideas, by their very nature,
must be speculative. I present them in the hope that they may illumi-
nate the distinction between the major life-threatening disease called
cancer and the far more ominous mask it usually wears. In order to
investigate this question, we must understand two psychological
concepts: the "shadow" and "projection."

The Disowned Self. Each of us would like to see himself in an
attractive light; honorable, generous, strong, sensitive and competent. We all at times think disagreeable thoughts, feel forbidden
desires and behave in ways that make us uncomfortable and
ashamed. We try to control these tendencies and are loath to acknowledge them in ourselves. But these unacceptable thoughts, feelings and forces do not just disappear. Rather, they become a hidden
part of ourselves, a part that Jung calls the *Shadow*.[51] The shadow can
include things we have never learned about ourselves and things
which we have some inkling of but would prefer not to know. We
try to keep our shadow side secret from the world and from ourselves. The admirable and demonic sides of a personality have been
portrayed in such stories as "Dr. Jekyll and Mr. Hyde." Each of us
has a subtle version of "Mr." or "Ms." Hyde dwelling within,
whether acknowledged or not.

The Process of Projection. Psychologists use the term *projection* to
describe the process of seeing in the outer world or in other people
that which is really inside of us. In much the same way that a movie
is projected onto a screen we project certain attitudes or feelings
onto people or places: "He hates me because this horrible thing is
growing in my body." "She doesn't love me because I can't provide
for her any more." "The children are disgusted by me since I have
become ill."

Projecting the Shadow. There is a grotesque historical instance of the projection of the shadow onto the enemy. "For over five years this man has been chasing around Europe like a madman in search of something he could set on fire. Unfortunately he again and again finds hirelings who open the gates of their country to this international incendiary."[52]

This quotation, which we well might expect to have been made about Adolf Hitler, is in fact from a speech Hitler made describing Winston Churchill. Although not on so global a scale, projection of this kind is quite common. A hidden, sinister, irrational, power-hungry intent is ascribed to the enemy as a means of locating odious tendencies "out there."

When the shadow is experienced, it is usually projected onto some external, recognizable form. An enemy serves as the perfect vehicle, but when a convenient enemy is not available, the form can be even more unexpected and frightening. The author Henry James, Sr., father of William and Henry James, describes such an experience in his autobiography.

> One day . . . towards the close of May, having eaten a comfortable dinner, I remained sitting at the table after the family had dispersed, idly gazing at the embers in the grate, thinking of nothing, and feeling only the exhilaration incident to a good digestion, when suddenly—in a lightning flash as it were—there came upon me, a rumbling which made all my bones to shake. To all appearance it was a perfectly insane and abject terror, without ostensible cause and only to be accounted for to my perplexed imagination, by some damned shape squatting invisible to me within the precincts of the room and raying out from his fetid personality influences fatal to life. The thing had not lasted 10 seconds before I felt myself a wreck; that is reduced from a state of firm, vigorous, joyful manhood to one of almost helpless infancy.[53]

This experience is vivid. Yet we all possess a shadow force and all have the potential to experience it. Since the shadow side of our personality can cause enormous anxiety, we all attempt to disown it. We do so, as we have seen, by projecting the shadow onto something "out there."

The many reports of strange "creature" sightings attest to this.

Recently a "large upright hairy creature" was vaguely seen by a few people in a small community. Everyone became terrified. Although it had never hurt anyone or even come close to anyone, it was pictured as a "sinister and dangerous beast." Several people shot at it; many others barricaded their doors and windows. It was spotted only at night and was perceived only as a blur, but dozens of men from neighboring communities came to hunt the "beast." The story became news when the local sheriff announced that the hunters were shooting at "every moving shadow" and might kill one another. He was alarmed that the hunt had taken on a "carnival atmosphere," with beer and transistor radios.[54]

Stories of this kind are not unusual and we must ask ourselves what is being hunted with such enthusiasm. In this case, the sheriff believed it was a bear. But a bear could not possibly provoke such a murderous assault. No one had seen the "creature" distinctly. No harm had been done. But the alleged "beast" served as a perfect physical manifestation of the shadow and as such inspired a crowd of hunters to destroy it.

But what has all this to do with our extreme fear of cancer? I believe that in many important respects the extra fear of cancer and the intense fear of the shadow are closely related. I believe that they are derived from the same psychological sources, and that the extra, intense fear associated with the image of cancer *is* the shadow which has been projected into it. Let me illustrate.

Cancer as a Shadow Form. The American Cancer Society describes cancer as follows: "For some unknown reason, one cell changes and begins to reproduce in a *wild* and *disorderly* way. They become *hungrier, steal* nourishment from their normal neighbors and *crowd them out.*"[55] A noted cancer specialist gives a similar portrait: "Cancer is one of the most *intractable,* variable and *incomprehensible* forms of cellular *derangement.* A cancer is a crab as its name indicates. It *claws* at us, it *hides* in the sands of our flesh; like a crab it *ignores straight walking,* progresses sideways both in its refusal to behave in an *honest,* purposeful manner, and in its need to *invade* neighboring tissues and to *shoot* some of its cells far away from its point of origin."[56] (Italics mine.)

How does it come about that words such as *wild, disorderly, hungrier* or *derangement* are used to portray an illness? How does it come about that phrases such as *refusal to behave in an honest manner, claws at us, steal nourishment from their normal neighbors,* or *hides in the sands of our flesh* are used to describe a disease? A scientific description of any disease can be unpleasant to read, but these descriptions portray more than illness. They are descriptions of a vicious and sinister enemy. Compare the following definition. "Cancer is a term used to indicate various types of malignant neoplasms, most of which are invasive, may metastasize to several sites and are likely to recur and cause death unless adequately treated."[57]

The last description concerns a disease process; the first two have much more to do with a sinister force which has been projected into a disease. We, as a culture, have made cancer a shadow form, a receptacle for our disowned self. This process is already evident in a twelve-year-old child's experience: "The reason I picked the theme Fight Cancer [in a poster contest] is because I see him as a dark and deadly monster. We don't know much about him nor can we predict what he'll do next or where he will strike or even whom he will strike."[58] This twelve-year-old girl is already prepared to experience the "extra" fear and "degradation" associated with cancer. She already expresses its imagery in terms of the dark and sinister force of the shadow. Is it not apparent, given this spontaneous imagery and constant cultural reinforcement, how easily the shadow might become synonymous with the image of cancer and then with the disease itself? Is it any wonder that a cancer patient would describe the experience of cancer as follows: "I feel so degraded, like a beast."[59]

Projection is such a habitual process that we effortlessly locate our shadow in the image of cancer. The image serves as an ideal form to represent those qualities we fear and loathe in ourselves. The *image* of cancer works perfectly as a means of separating ourselves from these qualities. But the mechanism of projection backfires once *cancer* has been diagnosed. The shadow-contaminated image then becomes rooted within us. Having projected our shadow into the image of cancer in order to disown it, we suffer the consequences of having it come back into us in the reality of the disease.

But cancer is only an illness; it is we who have taken what might have been the experience of a major disease and made it into a semi-conscious struggle with evil. Webster's Dictionary reflects this idea by listing "a source of evil" among its definitions of cancer. Let us pause for a moment to consider what other force once threatened us in a similar manner.

Before the age of enlightenment, most people believed in the Devil. He was the embodiment of evil. He was the source of all immoral tendencies, bad thoughts and dark deeds. What man wanted to disavow in himself was attributed to the Devil. When we became "enlightened" it was no longer possible to believe in so obvious an image or to deny responsibility in so obvious a manner. Citizens of a "modern" era, we embrace a rational, scientific view of life. And yet it may well be that we are on no friendlier terms with the evil in ourselves and no closer to accepting responsibility for it than we were when the Devil was to blame. For many of us today, cancer has come to be experienced with precisely the same terror the Devil inspired in our great grandparents.

It is no easy task to exorcise the demon from the image of cancer. We have experienced this dirty, dark, sinister image for many years. But if we see cancer as a group of diseases that afflict us in much the same way that other diseases afflict us, if we remember that many types of cancer are curable and few are totally resistant to some form of treatment, if we understand that this particular disease has become a vehicle for the shadow side of ourselves, we all stand a better chance of separating the experience of a potentially life-threatening disease from an ongoing private struggle with our disowned self. Experiencing the sinister image of cancer leads inevitably to a sense of despair, as if a statement had been whispered within: "I have been caught and will never escape." Cancer, on the other hand, viewed as presented in the above neutral, scientific passage, might well become another of the serious illnesses which afflict our lives but do not necessarily destroy us, fill us with horror or irreparably injure our sense of decency and self-worth. There are over 1,500,000 Americans who are very much alive and cured of this illness,[60] eloquent examples of the very different statement: "I was treated, cured and am now free of cancer."

2

Depression and Anger

I felt a strength flooding through me, lifting me from the depression of disappointment to a state of almost cheerful abandon. I felt the bitter aggression of the predator fill my mind.

—DOUGAL ROBERTSON, *Survive the Savage Sea*

Beneath the Wave of Despair

A vast amount of the *anxiety* experienced by cancer patients and their families is represented by terrifying images—images that fill the vacuum of unknowing. The majority of these fearful images are anticipatory: anxiety antecedent to expected loss. It is the dominant experience *prior* to cancer treatment. *Depression* is the predominant mood *following* it.[1] In many respects, anxiety is directed toward the future while depression reflects the past—threatened loss as compared with accomplished fact. But, as we have seen, "facts" are interpreted and it is the interpretation of these facts that evokes the most intense of responses.

Anxiety and depression represent almost polar moods. The experience of anxiety reflects the desire to survive; it is a force of life. But, if the instinct to survive is replaced by resignation, the mood of anxiety then converts to one of depression.[2] Depression and anxiety reflect opposing forces but they are not mutually exclusive. Many people experience states of anxious depression or alternating periods of anxiety and depression. "I'm so upset all the time, nervous and afraid to be alone. It's so stupid. I get furious at myself for being this way."[3] This woman is experiencing fear (afraid to be alone), anxiety (so upset all the time) and anger (furious at myself). She is not depressed, but these emotions can constellate a depression if they grow more intense. Beneath the restlessness, the fear and the rage is the sad, weary, self-condemning voice of depression. Another woman, lost in despair, says: "I feel so low. Why should I go on living?" And under this weary pronouncement might lurk the unacceptable and therefore banished anger, the unacknowledged anxiety and the suppressed will to survive.

Depression and anger reflect diverging but related emotional forces. Some people can more easily tolerate sadness and helplessness; others prefer the tension of angry confrontation. Anger often lies hidden below waves of despair; tears are often trapped behind barricades of anger. These conflicting tendencies toward anger and depression are closely bound to one another. Although complex, the dynamics of depression are certainly not beyond our capacity to comprehend. And, when we understand more fully what is happening in the depressed state, we are in a better position to *tolerate* what must be accepted and to *resolve* what is resolvable.

The Experience of Depression. We can experience both physical and emotional pain when depressed. People report aching joints, dizziness, nausea, stomach cramps and headaches. These symptoms persist despite the fact that diagnostic tests reveal no discernible cause. The common response, "it's only in the head," distorts the reality of depression; physical symptoms are present and pain experienced is real pain. Anguish, guilt, self-loathing, anger and helpless agitation can be even more difficult to bear. Depressed cancer patients often sit hopelessly, despairing how to go on. Everything about them slows down; their thinking, movement and conversation seem dull and obtuse. They often feel a burden to themselves and to others and therefore "remove" themselves by withdrawing into a painful isolation. Conversely, it is not easy to feel responsible for someone who is depressed. Family members can become frustrated and resentful; some begin to feel depressed themselves. Thoughts of suicide are not infrequent and should not be taken lightly despite the fact that actual suicide by cancer patients is extremely rare.[4] The idea of suicide, whether acted on or not, reveals despair and desperate need. This is especially true when the spouse of a cancer patient is depressed. A former director of the suicide prevention society states: "When dealing with cancer related stress, we receive relatively few calls from cancer patients. The majority . . . are either the spouse or a relative of the cancer patient."[5] Severe depression can affect anyone involved with the cancer experience.

Convincing Mood of Self-Deception. Depressions can be characterized as "retarded" or "agitated." There is a dramatic decrease in activity with the *retarded* type. The person is not only dejected but prefers to stay still, speak very little and have nothing asked of him: "They don't seem to understand that I just can't do anything, I can't even think of anything, it's all over."[6] Everything seems hopeless; there is constant sadness and a conviction of being worthless. When the depression takes the form of *agitated* activity, the gloomy mood of self-contempt is the same, but rather than sitting in silent postures of despair, those afflicted cannot keep still. They move constantly, have difficulty getting rest or sleep, are often unable to slow down their racing thoughts and pace back and forth like caged criminals.

When any of us are gripped by depression, it is rarely possible to see past the depressed mood. The sense of oneself is severely disturbed, perceptions are self-condemning, the inner voice mocking and self-disparaging. A beauty queen is referred to me by a plastic surgeon because she is sure that her face is repulsive. A successful scientist seeks therapy because he is convinced that he is stupid and has only temporarily deceived his colleagues. No amount of evidence to the contrary can alter these sweeping convictions. The depressive mood insists on its own reality. Perceptions filtered through such a depressed mood are violent distortions, small fragments of the unobserved whole, self-contemptuous proclamations disguised as realistic assessment. However, the awareness that one's self-contempt, despair and helplessness are not newly discovered facts but rather symptoms of depression becomes apparent only after the depression has lifted. I offer the same counsel to those with whom I work that I do to myself when depressed: "Do not believe the inner voice of depression; it is a cunning master of self-deceit. Do not take the condemnations to heart; they are symptoms and not legitimate conclusions. Remember that although it is difficult to see beyond a depressed mood, depressions do end."

Amoral Origins. The "endogenous" depression (internally generated) is closely related to body chemistry. A perfect example is post-partum depression. A young mother feels sad and withdrawn after giving birth rather than happy and enthusiastic as she had expected. Her depression is profoundly confusing. She has dreamed and planned for her baby with tender anticipation and then experiences great sadness. A large part of the depression has to do with the physical changes occurring in her body. Every woman's glandular metabolism is affected by pregnancy and birth. But, for some, metabolic changes exceed their nervous system's tolerance and a woman then experiences the symptoms of depression.[7] These symptoms make it easy for her to conclude that she is a shamefully unfit mother. To the outsider, the self-condemning assessment is unduly harsh. What is shameful about emotional symptoms that result from a temporary imbalance of the nervous system? But if you have experienced a post-partum depression, you know that no one can talk you out of your self-condemnations until the depression has lifted.

Endogenous depression of this kind regularly affects cancer patients. Surgery, radiation therapy and chemotherapy have enormous impact on body chemistry. Internal systems become temporarily imbalanced: "Dad doesn't eat very much and he seems to be awake all the time. I don't even know if he is in pain—he hardly talks. But he seems so sad and low."[8] Depression of this kind can occur during hospitalization and following discharge, when a great deal of energy is required for physical recuperation and there is little reserve for the many psychological demands of this time. It can also occur whenever there is long-term stress whether for patient or family member. It is possible for family members to exceed their body's physical and emotional capacities, to neglect their personal needs for rest and sustenance and to become exhausted through overidentification with the patient. Depression will often follow such extreme effort.

The endogenous depression derives from biochemical changes within the body. However, depression based on emotional conflict can accompany it. A post-partum depression also illustrates this phenomenon. In addition to the hormonal imbalance inherent in pregnancy and birth, there is often underlying conflict and doubt. A new mother might be afraid she will not know how to raise a child; she feels happy that the baby is healthy and angry because of all the new responsibility. Conflict of this sort can produce another kind of depression, a depressed mood that issues from intense emotional discord. Are we to judge physical stress and hormonal imbalance as a more worthy source of depression than emotional conflict? Are we to sympathize with bodily exhaustion and disdain one of the most common sources of conflict: to support the new mother wholeheartedly only if her depression does not result from emotional discord? It would seem cruel and arbitrary, and yet many of us judge ourselves in precisely this way.

Cancer treatment can cause far greater *physical* stress than pregnancy and birth. It is therefore not surprising that it causes depression. Cancer treatment also evokes much more anxiety, anger, doubt and conflict than a newborn baby and it is therefore not at all surprising that cancer patients are afflicted with depressive moods that derive from these *nonphysical* sources as well. The physical impact of surgery, radiation therapy and chemotherapy is self-evident and can simply overload the nervous system. Depressive symptoms will then emerge and many will subside as the body recuperates. But the conflicts and doubts and outrages (the emotional sources of depression) can be more obscure and more difficult to deal with.

The Last Straw and Achilles Heel. Some depressions are derived from accumulated stress. The "straw that broke the camel's back" is a perfect image for this kind of experience. To those of us who feel as if we have had to endure a great many tribulations and are therefore just barely staying ahead of life's demands, cancer treatment might be easily experienced as the "last straw." There is, however, another experience of depression. To those of us who have made an unusually strong investment in specific activities or in specific physical attributes, cancer treatment might easily be experienced as an alarming threat. The "Achilles heel" image captures the correct sense of this kind of vulnerability.

The presence of an "Achilles heel" and the degree of associated vulnerability depend on the internal mental picture each of us has of himself. Surgery changes the body in conspicuous ways, yet depression more often proceeds from what the affected part symbolized. For example, no one likes to lose his hair, but if hair represents strength and masculinity (as it did for Samson) then the blow to one's self-image is extreme. It is the meaning contained in the symbol of baldness that causes the grim preoccupation with hair loss. Cancer surgery also results in this kind of symbolic loss and produces related depression. Consider the general symbolic categories. The face often represents our identity. When placed on passports or licenses the picture says "This is who I am." Surgery to the head and neck areas threatens to strip away an identity; our despair issues from symbolically having "lost face." Breasts and genitals are more than functional organs. Loss or disfigurement of them carries shame and the fear of rejection. A small biopsy of the breast, although benign and not at all disfiguring, can trigger depression. The loss is symbolic but the depression can be as intense as when radical surgery has been performed. Cleanliness, proper behavior and the ability to control oneself are often identified with the rectum. The loss of normal bowel function can have a devastating impact on one's self-image and self-esteem. Legs represent independence, hands stand for skill and accomplishment.[9] All carry great symbolic meaning and all can therefore cause great distress when injured or lost.

The Driving Force of Depression

A simple explanation of depression involves energy. If too much physiological energy is consumed in physical and emotional stress, the resulting chronic fatigue causes an "exhaustion of adaptive energy."[10] In this simple system, the symptoms of depression are the experiences of "exhausted adaptability." But the forces of depression are more specific than the image of fatigue would suggest.

Freud was the first to clarify the underlying themes. By tracing the experiences of emptiness, loss of interest and physical depletion to the process of grief, he was able to separate and describe the different mechanism of depression. He found that it comprised feelings of inadequacy, unworthiness, powerlessness and self-loathing: the devastating feelings that accompany the loss of self-esteem. These experiences are not the product of grief but rather the inevitable consequences of anger directed against oneself.[11] This dynamic is now widely accepted as an explanation for the incredible driving force of depression. The inner voice of the depressed man addresses himself in cruel, harsh, vindictive and condemning tones. We would not address another human being in such a harsh, judgmental manner. Both the principles of logic and the wisdom of compassion recommend kindness and generosity during times of stress. But the depressed person feels he deserves neither kindness nor generosity, and the driving force of this condemning voice is rage. "They all looked like goddamned fools. My daughter got sick and she died and they never even knew what was wrong with her. There is this enormous fifteen-floor institution with thousands of people and yet they seemed so small, like such fools. That's when I just gave up. I thought, shit, if they don't know, I guess there is just no answer. My anger dissolved. I really got morose, I went way down. [*Why do you think you gave up?*] There was so much rage. I could have pulled my hair out or beat my face against a wall and I thought, my God, I can't even get an answer to one little question—what's wrong with her? I lost all hope, there was nothing to hold on to. [*You don't seem like someone who gives up easily.*] Do you see how angry I get when I start to talk about it, how I start building up? It's still all inside but back then I just let go."[12]

The frustration of the three following fundamental aspirations often leads to outrage and depression. The desire to be *loved and respected,* the wish to be *strong and superior,* the resolve to be *good and loving*[13] are different in kind and yet can easily coexist in varying combinations within each of us. We aspire to achieve these goals and, if achieved, we aspire to maintain the resulting status. But if thwarted a person feels frustrated and angry, directs the anger against himself, suffers a loss of self-esteem and becomes depressed.

To Be Loved and Respected. Many of us share a secret shame and a secret fear of being exposed. We spend a lifetime trying to overcome our doubts and fears, a lifetime trying to hide them from others, endeavoring to establish a feeling of personal worthiness that can justify being loved and respected. For many people, the diagnosis of cancer is experienced as "being found out," as having "something wrong," as the end of feeling "worthy." All too often a person who has been plagued by the shameful thought "if only they knew" begins, after cancer treatment, to draw the shameful conclusion "now they know." The wish to be loved and respected then seems beyond reach and a depressed mood emerges. The tragedy of this process is that it has almost nothing to do with the disease we call cancer or its treatment. It emerges from the patient's personal interpretation of what cancer means. Being loved and respected obviously has much more to do with how one behaves than with what diseases afflict one's body. However, if a cancer patient becomes convinced that he is no longer worthy of love and respect, he will often begin to behave in a manner calculated to provoke rejection, and he will then bitterly conclude that he was right all along.

Members of a cancer patient's family can also trap themselves in this particular process of depression: "Jim is the only man who has ever really known me. I can be myself with him and he still loves me. If he dies, I am sure I'll never have that again."[14] "Suppose she dies before I can show her that I'm someone she can be proud of. Maybe there's not enough time. She'll never know, never really believe in me. She'll never be able to really give me her blessing because I won't have made it before she's gone."[15] Here too the need to be worthy of love and respect is threatened by the diagnosis of cancer. Family members are often angry at the cancer patient for being ill and jeopardizing an important source of their love and self-esteem. They deny or condemn the anger, experience guilt about this "inappropriate feeling" and in turn become depressed.

To Be Strong and Superior. Many of us aspire to be dominant, to feel strong and in command, to be better than anyone else. Some of us have achieved this goal; others maintain a seemingly realistic hope that one day they will feel securely "on top of things." The diagnosis and treatment of cancer can be experienced as a stinging blow to such aspirations of strength and superiority. The shock comes from interpreting the cancer as evidence (whether actual, imaginary or symbolic) that one's "underlying weakness" has won: "I've been betrayed by my body. Now I'm trapped and must suffer my fate. There is no way I can fight it. I don't have any weapons to use . . . how can I defeat what I can't even get my hands on? Maybe I've just kidded myself for a long time."[16] This man had thrived on competition and challenge. He had always scorned inactivity and driven himself upward. His self-esteem was founded on a "gladiator" image and his striving to be the best at whatever he did. He became enraged at the cancer and marched into battle to defeat it. But the treatment dragged on. He could not accept the "damned timidness" of his doctors and could not quite trust them. His rage and disappointment were finally turned against himself and he became extremely depressed. He began to say: "There is no way I can really make it any more. I've just given up." This man's bitter depression did not derive from feeling unlovable. It arose from the fact that he could no longer esteem himself as a conquering hero. All alternative possibilities were wholly unacceptable, for he would not consider any suggestion that was less than his unyielding wish for dominance and superiority.

The same process occurs with family members. A wife or husband, parent or child who regularly assume responsibility for the problems of others by trying to "make everything all right" will often experience a great loss of power and effectiveness during the cancer crisis. The illusion of potential omnipotence can be stubbornly maintained despite our knowledge that its attainment is impossible. Depression will often attend this frustrated but persistent aspiration to be strong enough to make everything all right for a loved one.

To Be Good and Loving. Many of us aspire to be truly generous, to love without the contamination of selfish desires or ulterior motives, to experience ourselves as free from pettiness or hostility. If we discover an inner anger or a streak of meanness, we condemn ourselves and suffer a dramatic loss of self-esteem. The diagnosis and treatment of cancer always stimulates anger whether we approve of it or not, and this experience of anger can be extremely unwelcome. When the justifiable anger of the cancer experience is disowned or denied, it becomes transformed into depression.[17] It is, in fact, the most common source of depression, and we would profit from taking the time to explore thoroughly the many possible sources of anger associated with cancer and to examine in detail what can happen when the anger is badly managed.

Behind the Barricade of Anger

Almost all physically healthy people maintain an illusion of invulnerability; we strive to maintain an inner certainty that, while others may fall, we will be spared. The diagnosis of cancer shatters these vaguely held feelings of invulnerability and most of us violently protest its loss. The bitter protest continues to rage within us when the diagnosis does not change. A few people experience the rage for years: "The frustration and anger, after all this time, is like a magnet. Sometimes you really don't want to care but you're drawn back to it, to a point where you can't keep away and you've got to do something."[18]

Searching for Specific Targets. Anger can always find a target: "My son Bobby kept slapping at me. I'd tell him not to hit so hard and he'd scream, 'They're doing it to me.' We got him a punching clown and he beat the hell out of it."[19] Cancer or death can be experienced as a hated enemy: "It's been eight years since my son was diagnosed and I'm still pissed off that the whole goddamned thing happened. Somebody saying your son has cancer, this beautiful child is going to die just because of this crummy disease." "I hate those who make death sound so romantic. That's such crap. It's an ugly, horrible thing to face and no supposedly proper attitude is going to change that."[20]

More often, however, the anger is directed at others, and although rarely aware of it, physicians are often the primary targets. I have never attended a conference for cancer patients or for the families of cancer patients without hearing endless bitter complaints directed at the medical profession. Many conflicts concern the tone and manner in which the diagnosis and treatment plan were discussed. Many reflect the boiling hatred reserved for the messenger of evil tidings. However, most grievances are more specific: the doctor was negligent, incompetent, cursory, impersonal. Some of the charges have to do with the physician's destruction of hope. Other patients resent unfulfilled promises: "He kept saying just hang in there and everything will be fine. And I did. Everyone was so proud of me. But he lied and it's not fair. I don't think I would have consented to surgery if I had known. All of this misery comes from having trusted him."[21] Since so much authority is granted to the physician, intense rage attends his limits, inabilities, well-meaning deceptions, oversights and mistakes.

In a study of parents at one of the largest cancer centers in the United States,[22] it was a rare occurrence to find a mother who was not enraged with the doctors. I have found the same burning resentments: "I thought that medicine and leukemia were like *Medical Center* or *Dr. Welby.* Then I found that people look the other way, they duck around corners. I was absolutely horrified and furious. . . . If only one doctor had said 'How are you doing?' " "I lost my father two years ago . . . he died of cancer and the medical profession botched on that. They really goofed it up. I tried to tell myself, 'They're not gods,' I tried to rationalize but I'm still furious for what happened." "I know what it's about, how grossly you can be treated. Before I went through it I would have seriously doubted the perspective I have now. I would have thought it was a lot of grumbling over nothing. Then I saw it in action and how gross the doctors can be."[23]

These grievances are rarely expressed to the physician. Family members, nurses and many others more often hear the bitter out-bursts: "I yelled at David a lot. I'd scream, 'Don't bother to come home.' I didn't mean it, but said it anyway. I wasn't proud of my-self." "When Peter was very sick, he insisted his brother Michael give him the shot. He'd say to him, 'You're not going to get away completely.' He was furious because Michael was going to live and he made him be a part of his illness." "I was the most exasperated with the hospital chaplain. When he said, 'God gives burdens to those who can carry them.' Hell, is that true for all those people jumping off the bridge?" "There was my mother, this dignified, proud old woman. And the nurses, I could have killed them. 'Okay, dearie, do this. C'mon, honey, roll over now.' Did they think they were talking to a dog? My God, I could just have killed them."[24]

Possibly the most painful anger to bear is that directed at a sick child: ". . . when she got sick she changed my whole life. Admitting that I was angry at my own baby was horrible. . . . That she was ripping off my life and relationship to my husband."[25]

Most of these statements were made in retrospect, after the anger had partially subsided. Most were made in a supportive and sympa-thetic environment. Anger can be extremely difficult to experience and express without shame and guilt.

Lost Integrity and Willing Victims. It is a fact worthy of attention that the experience and expression of anger are regarded with such abhorrence. Anger is as natural and universal an experience as love, hunger, sadness, sexuality or fatigue. *All of us* get angry just as predictably as all of us get hungry. However, many of us will allow ourselves to experience only those emotions we designate as socially acceptable and express only those emotions we believe to be socially attractive. Anger is one of the first emotions to be banished.

The suppression of anger is not restricted to cancer patients. Stud-ies show the tendency to be alarmingly widespread. In one study, entitled "A Nation of Willing Victims," researchers found that most people were willing to tolerate outrageous personal insults in their attempts to avoid confrontations. They obtained a consistent result with a variety of social provocations: "The great majority of subjects (over 80 percent) proved willing victims when others violated their rights."[26] Why are we such willing victims? What overriding consideration makes most of us passively accept these affronts, refuse to honor our personal integrity or respect our personal rights? What is there about anger that makes the status of victim preferable to admitting that we don't like being victimized? The larger social questions are complex and not the immediate concern of this work. But the more specific question of anger and cancer is of immediate concern to us.

The diagnosis and treatment of cancer evoke rage, the sense of losing control and fear of rejection. It is the rage which leads to the fear of causing offense and thereby losing the support and sympathy of others. In the emerging conflict between the rage and the magnified need for affectionate support, anger can be easily turned against oneself and lead to depression. This seems to be less true of cardiac patients. Well-known studies portray them as quite rebellious and thereby less burdened with suppressed anger.[27] But the widespread occurrence of guilty repentance among cancer patients suggests that cancer carries an additional injunction against expressed anger. By feeling they "haven't the right" to be angry, cancer patients create another pathway toward depression. For some of us, even the actual experience of anger can create a fear of losing control. This occurs when one believes that to get mad is to be mad, that to get angry is kin to going crazy. Although expressing anger is the very antithesis of madness, the fear persists that losing control through the expression of anger will lead to mental imbalance. Being angry may not fit the desire to be constantly loving, but there is a great deal of healthy ground between sainthood and the mental ward. And there is certainly a place for anger in the cancer experience.

Physical Consequences of Denied Anger. I have illustrated the depressive symptoms of denied anger. There are physical consequences as well. Imagine someone you know who is angry and will not admit it. He can rarely disguise all signs: lips tighten and jaw muscles bulge, the skin gets redder or it blanches, breathing becomes more rapid, at times there is puffiness in the neck and face or the eyes visibly harden. Over a longer period of time, the internal consequences of unexpressed anger can be injurious, especially when disease is present. Diabetics find it much easier to maintain control of their disease by means of medication when they are able to express anger.[28] Cancer patients who tend to be the most eager to please others, those who deny themselves a productive form of emotional expression, have been shown to suffer proportionally faster tumor growth.[29]

For many years, cancer patients were considered nonparticipating bystanders while their tumor received the physicians' full attention. It is now becoming increasingly apparent that complex *physical and emotional* forces contribute to the success or failure of medical treatment. Who we are and how we behave *influence* cancer treatment and recovery. It is impossible to determine exact degrees of influence but it is relatively easy to establish the presence of influence, especially during recuperation.

Several years ago I evaluated the post-treatment progress of forty-five cancer patients.[30] They varied in their degree of surgical impairment and in their abilities to adjust to the cancer crisis. All were free of any evidence of disease. I was searching for factors which tended to influence the success of adjustment. Two distinct groups emerged from a comprehensive one-year follow-up evaluation; the members of one group were experiencing great difficulty reestablishing their lives; the members of another group were doing so with much less difficulty. It is interesting to note that the majority of those who experienced the greatest adjustment problems were rated as particularly "unassertive." Disowned and unexpressed anger were shown to be characteristic of those who were less able to deal with the emotional and physical stress of cancer treatment. Such obvious factors as age and the degree of surgical impairment showed no correlation with adjustment success. We must therefore ask this crucial question: Are there alternatives for those of us who are victimized by powerful prohibitions against the expression of anger? The answer is yes.

Anger Petty and Anger Heroic. The first task is to alter our perspective in regard to anger. Let us listen to one thoughtful man struggling with this question: "Always I turn away from anger as petty and mean, destructive of life, and so it is often, but not always. There is another kind of anger, different in quality, in implication, in consequence; when one beholds it one sees nothing ugly but something grand. . . . It knows nothing of meanness or spite; it is the passion of the doer who will not let his work be swept aside. It hurts no one, it asserts life, it is the force that generates form. Its opposite is not love but weakness . . . in danger I will feel either fear or anger and either may be self-preserving. If I am to avoid danger by running, fear will help me run faster; if I am to stand my ground, anger will help me stand it more firmly."[31] This sense of anger serves the best in each of us.

A vivid description of how anger can literally sustain life is contained in the documented account of a shipwrecked family's struggle to survive. During the seventh day on a life raft in the mid-Pacific with little water and their morale at low ebb, they finally sighted a cargo ship and began to celebrate their anticipated rescue. The father set off hand flares when the ship was within three miles of them. It seemed unimaginable to him that some crewman could fail to see his distress signals spiraling through the sky. But the ship sailed slowly by and disappeared over the horizon. "I surveyed the empty flare cartons bitterly . . . and something happened to me in that instant that for me changed the whole aspect of our predicament. If those poor bloody seamen couldn't rescue us then we would have to make it on our own and to hell with them. . . . I felt a strength flooding through me, lifting me from the depression of disappointment to a state of almost cheerful abandon. I felt the bitter aggression of the predator fill my mind."[32] The family did survive. They stayed afloat and lived off the sea for thirty-eight long days and were finally rescued. The turning-away from despair and the emergence of a cunning instinct for survival would not have been possible without the father's passionate anger. Honest anger in the service of physical or spiritual self-preservation is never petty or ugly.

I want to stress the crucial difference between expressing anger and acting on aggressive feelings. If we believe that anger must inevitably lead to destructive fighting we will naturally condemn anger. But if we can realize that the honest expression of anger results in less injury to others and to ourselves, we will then be in a better position to accept it as one of the universal experiences of life. The ability to forgive and forget is essential to any healthy relationship. Angry feelings must be experienced and expressed before genuine forgiveness can be offered and accepted.

The inability to experience one's anger leads to diminished physical resistance and the symptoms of depression. But the ability to tolerate the *experience* of anger is a step toward wholeness. One is able to make contact with feelings, with possible modes of expression, with alternative choices and with a sense of personal authority.

The *expression* of anger is a positive and healthy process. All of us —patient, family member, nurse or physician—must try to be as accepting of this emotion as we possibly can be. The hope of uninterrupted harmony is a destructive ideal; it must generate unresolvable emotional conflict. The acceptance of anger is a far more productive aspiration and may well comprise one of the fundamental tasks of our humanity.

The Road Back. We may countenance the process of depression by proclaiming ourselves worthless individuals or we may nourish the process of recovery by discovering a personal task and tolerating the anger and anxiety that are an essential part of its achievement. We are all free to define and redefine our goals. This is an especially important task during the cancer crisis. It can elevate self-esteem, which in turn fosters an inner opposition to the rabid voice of self-condemnation. Anger is redirected and a feeling of personal authority begins to emerge, despair and frustration recede, hopelessness fades and alternative choices become more apparent. These phases of recovery have been called the "process of restitution."[33] They require an understanding and an acceptance of the fact that we create our own emotional reality. The process of restitution is possible; the depression associated with the cancer crisis is resolvable. To relinquish an ideal is always painful, but the claiming of one's humanity through acts of self-acceptance makes us vigorous actors in our own destiny rather than the passive and despairing victims of our fate.

3

The Work of Mourning

Give sorrow words. The grief that does not speak
Whispers the o'er-frought heart and bids it break.
—SHAKESPEARE

The loss of anything valued or of anyone loved inevitably leaves a terrible wound. Emotional healing takes place through the process of mourning. The experience of grief is universally experienced and yet hard to portray. Social scientists describe symptoms: "There is apt to be an aching tightness in the throat, sometimes a choking sensation, shortness of breath and a frequent need for sighing, all of these being related to a feeling of wanting to cry . . . a feeling of weakness and easy exhaustion."[1] Only poets have been able to capture some of the essence of this intense bittersweet emotion:

Grief tears his heart, and drives him to and fro.
In all the raging impotence of woe.
(ALEXANDER POPE)

By the waters of the woodland
I have looked for you
Weeping in the meadow I lay down
I light the lamps of my heart.
I call your name
From the deeps of the world
From the hollow place
You do not come.

What hath become of you?
My lad. My lovely one.
                        (KIM CHERNIN)

Home they brought her warrior dead;
    She nor swoon'd nor utter'd cry.
All her maidens, watching, said,
    "She must weep or she will die."

Then they praised him, soft and low,
    Call'd him worthy to be loved,
Truest friend and noblest foe;
    Yet she neither spoke nor moved.

Stole a maiden from her place,
    Lightly to the warrior stept,
Took the face-cloth from his face;
    Yet she neither moved nor wept.

Rose a nurse of ninety years,
    Set his child upon her knee—
Like summer tempest came her tears—
    "Sweet, my child, I live for thee."
                        (ALFRED TENNYSON)

Child, parent, husband or wife, dream, ability, possession or goal: grief attends the loss of anyone loved or anything valued. Unspoken grief bids the heart to break, yet the princess of Tennyson's poem, like so many of us, had first "neither moved nor wept." Mourning is at once both a natural and an inexpressibly painful process. It should also be thought of as extremely difficult work. The work of mourning can be as important as any single aspect of the cancer experience.

Some years ago I saw a woman who had just undergone extensive cancer surgery. Marsha was a strong and disciplined person, proud of her evident courage, deserving of the praise her husband and doctors bestowed upon her. Her pride helped her to fight back the tears she refused to acknowledge. I had spoken earlier with her husband. His face, a strained mask of resolute determination, betrayed no trace of sadness. Both husband and wife wanted only to know what was expected of them. Both were determined to "take care of business." When I was alone with Marsha, I asked her if she allowed herself to cry. She quickly replied that her husband would not be able to bear it. I told her that I was sorry that he, as yet, could not permit himself to cry and that I hoped he soon would be able to do so, but that I believed she was neglecting some important "business" of her own by refusing to mourn the many losses she had recently suffered. She wrapped her arms tightly around herself and began to tremble visibly. I said it seemed at this moment that she was feeling a great deal of sadness. Her shoulders shook, her eyes filled with tears and then, no longer restrained, her grief burst forth. She cried for over an hour, and when her weeping subsided, she looked at me with a somewhat bewildered expression and said: "With all my sadness, how can I be feeling uplifted?" But there is no mystery. Her face, which had seemed like a tight mask just an hour before, had become soft and human again. The tears that oppressed her with their accumulated weight were momentarily spent. Her experience of release and lightness was understandable and quite apparent. Crying is the first step in the expression of grief. Tears bear eloquent testimony to sorrow long before the right words can be found.

We, as a culture, have done a disservice to ourselves and to our loved ones by rewarding the ability to control disruptive emotion with great admiration. We have managed to cripple the work of mourning. Widows rarely wear black, men seldom wear mourning bands. The mourner cannot be recognized and is expected to become quickly reabsorbed in the activities of life. By minimizing the feelings and rituals of bereavement we have undermined an essential mode of healing.

Intense grief is an unwelcomed experience; it can evoke strong feelings of helplessness, fear, guilt and defeat. It is not surprising that we attempt to minimize it. Bereavement is not an easy or speedy task. In fact, it takes far more courage and strength to be open to the work of mourning, to be willing to experience one's vulnerability, actually to walk among the sufferers, than it does to erect a fortress of emotional armor around one's heart and remain forever hidden behind its protective barricades. It is certainly not necessary to involve ourselves in dramatic public grieving. But I believe that, public or private, shared with others or known only to the one who suffers, the experience of grief and the painful work of mourning are essential to the preservation of a rich and meaningful existence. The unmourned loss can haunt one's life and cause an experience of inexplicably bitter sadness. Anything lost must be accepted and mourned before it is possible to honor a loved memory and begin a new chapter of life. The process of grief can replenish each of us if we will but entrust ourselves to its healing powers.

Legacy of Loss

The diagnosis of cancer, in itself, constitutes the first loss. A healthy person is suddenly seriously ill and the shock of the diagnosis is followed by grief for the loss of good health. In time, a variety of hopes and expectations might also be lost and each calls for renewed grieving. These losses can include physical disfigurement or bodily impairment; loss of job, income or financial security; diminished social status or physical vitality; and one day, the most painful loss of all, the death of a loved one or the anticipation of one's own death and everything we value in life. Anticipated loss can involve other things as well. Some of us might feel grief for the "life never lived," others for underdeveloped personal qualities—tenderness in the authoritarian, daring in the more timid, accomplishment in the less ambitious. Grief attends the fear that sufficient time is no longer available to live the unlived life or to develop the dormant qualities of heart and mind.

The loss of a loved one carries an infinite number of meanings. Dickens describes this beautifully through an old man's memories of a young sailor thought to be drowned at sea. "Where's that young school boy with the rosy face and curly hair, that used to be as merry in this here parlor . . . as a piece of music? Gone down with Wal'r. Where's that there fresh lad, that nothing couldn't tire nor put out, and that sparkled up and blushed so when we joked about him, about Hearts Delight, that he was beautiful to look at? Gone down with Wal'r. Where's that there man's spirit, all afire, that wouldn't see the old man hove down for a moment, and cared nothing for itself?

Gone down with Wal'r. There was a dozen Wal'r that I knowed and loved, all holding round his neck when he went down, and there a holding around mine now."[2]

A woman describes similar remorse following the death of her husband: ". . . love without its object shrivels like a flower betrayed by an early frost. How can we live without it? This explains the passionate grief of widowhood. Grief is as much a lament for the end of love as anything else . . . [but] acceptance finally comes. And with it comes peace."[3]

The relinquishment of anything valued or anyone loved is extraordinarily painful. For many, it can be even more forbidding than the anticipation of death itself. In the Greek legend, Philemon and Baucis are granted one wish from the gods, and the lovers ask to die at the same moment. Not surviving a loved one, not experiencing the pain of loss, can be valued above all else. "Charlie and Josephine had been inseparable companions for thirteen years. In a senseless act of violence, Charlie, in full view of Josephine, was shot and killed in a melee with the police. Josephine first stood motionless, then slowly approached his prostrate form, sank to her knees, and silently rested her head on the dead and bloody body. Concerned persons attempted to help her away, but she refused to move. Hoping she would soon surmount her overwhelming grief, they let her be. But she never rose again, in fifteen minutes she was dead. . . . Charlie and Josephine were llamas in the zoo."[4]

The same choice is made by soldiers during the stress of war. It was a common occurrence for the crew of a bomber to go down with the crippled plane rather than abandon a wounded crewman.[5] The experience of loss and abandonment can be almost unbearable. Even a renowned social scientist, an expert on the importance of mourning, reports how she was unwilling to experience her husband's death and denied over and over again her feelings of grief. It was not until a close friend was accidentally killed that she began her work of mourning. "This news completely overwhelmed me; it was as if my carefully maintained defenses against breaking down could not withstand the shock. I collapsed helplessly and then did all the crying, expressed all the grief which really belonged to the loss of my husband."[6]

Ambivalence and Guilt

Difficulty performing the work of mourning is especially characteristic of those who have feelings of ambivalence about their bodies, occupations, roles in life, relationships or right to experience fulfillment. Excessive guilt and pronounced conflict will tend to shut down the process of grief. A man who yearned to be a novelist but was afraid to try in earnest lost his left eye because of cancer surgery. He became withdrawn and refused to consider further efforts at writing. "It serves me right for trying to be such a big shot," he said. "You see, an eye for an eye. Just try to see into things now. [*Are you sad or angry about the surgery?*] I got what I deserved. The big shot got put in his place, he was getting too big for his britches."[7] This man's interpretation of the loss of his eye is clear. The aspiration to be a novelist was forbidden; the punishment for transgression was one eye. There are many possible interpretations for his words, but for the purpose of this discussion, we note that he could not grieve the loss of that which he insisted was "just payment" for his shameful presumption, and he became depressed.

Couples who have fought long and bitter battles, those who have deceived one another for years and those who have never expressed their hidden resentments will experience lessened abilities to mourn. They tend to conclude that their previous feelings or actions deprive them of this universal human right. Neglecting the work of mourning commonly results in a feeling of detachment and sad purposelessness, a despair that can impoverish one's life. Following his wife's death in 1755, Boswell described this state of alienation: "I have ever since seemed to myself broken off from mankind; a kind of solitary wanderer in the wild of life, without any direction or fixed point of view; a gloomy gazer on the world to which I have little relation."[8]

The Solitude of Bereavement

The hard work of mourning brings pain, relief and finally peace. There is no other way to heal the terrible wound of loss or to renew life. The hardest part, for many of us, is the solitude of grief. In fact, the absence or unwillingness of others to share in one's grief can constitute still another loss. A cancer patient says: "Their [his family's] desire was always to hear from me that I was all right. . . . They never have the patience to listen to the whole story of my illness."9 A widow says: "When I'm really lonely, I often talk to a picture of us, taken on vacation, in a gold frame. This time I felt so sad and began to weep . . . then I saw that the gold on George's side was running. I swear I was not just seeing things. The gold ran down the frame, it was on my fingers. I kept saying to him: 'Don't cry, George, I'll be all right. Don't cry, my darling, I can make it.' I've never cried like that before or felt him so close since he died."10

The loneliness of grief is often experienced by children. In fact, many parents intentionally isolate their children in the hope of protecting them from unnecessary pain and distress. Unfortunately, this strategy usually places the uninformed child in the vulnerable position of trying to explain the inexplicable.

My parents did not know how carefully I had observed the course of my sister's illness and death. My mother's constant struggle was to keep me unaware, to protect me from the shadow of this personal tragedy that had fallen upon us . . . [But] I knew then, when my sister was dying, that something dreadful, ultimate and irreversible was going on. I may not have grasped the meaning of the word death, I may have been, at the age of five, incapable of the concept. But that there was, in our house, something too dreadful for words—that fact did not escape me. . . .

Few people ever overcome the anguish of the knowledge of death, no matter the age at which it enters into their life. But when a small child lives it, with all that strength and urgency of feeling so characteristic of childhood, very little that follows later in life will equal in intensity the dreadful sense of outrage and helpless impotence one feels as one lies there, aware of what is occurring with all one's senses: seeing it, hearing it, even smelling it, while all the time willing it not to happen, begging whatever powers there are in the universe to oppose it, to gather themselves against it, to forestall it and turn it back.

You try so many things, as a small child, a little believer in magic: you offer yourself in her place, you promise never to tell lies again, you swear never to be angry at anyone or to think bad thoughts. You pray and wish and will and command and bargain. You figure out solutions, you invent causes, you derive consequences from antecedent occurrences, you build, with feeling and passion, a world of metaphysical enquiry profoundly binding upon your future development.[11]

Feeling isolated with one's pain, whether as child or adult, can intensify loneliness and despair, but the experience of grief generates its own healing potential. It cannot be relieved by the presence of others.[12] Grief, like any other distress, is easier to endure when love and sympathetic support are available, but it must be endured.

I know of no more beautiful example of the universal need to grieve and the benefit of sympathetic understanding than that involving a seven-year-old mentally retarded boy. One morning he greeted his teacher tensely and showed her his new oversized wrist watch. When she had him make clay figures, as was their custom, he formed what seemed to be a coffin. Then, with great concentration, he made a heavy lid, picked up a hammer and smashed it onto the coffin with all his strength. When the teacher asked about this behavior he began to howl and throw himself about the room as if in great pain. Her inquiries led to the discovery that the boy's father had died the week before. He repeated the coffin ritual for the next six days. The teacher would admire his new watch and add that he must be so proud because it had been his daddy's, he would smile and nod his head, sit down, make a coffin and place a lid on top of it. The only difference was that each day the lid grew lighter and it was placed on the coffin with greater care. On the seventh day, he made a very thin lid, placed it gently on the coffin and made several holes in it. The teacher commented, "That's right. Now your daddy can breathe." The boy smiled with evident relief at her understanding. The following day he again made a coffin, looked at it for a moment and built it into a basket. He then made clay fruit to fill it.[13]

The Healing Process of Grief

This young boy had accomplished the work of mourning in his own way. He had expressed rage and pain, and with his teacher's kind understanding, he had made peace with his father's death. All of us can learn a profound lesson from this child: we must feel what we feel, express it in our own way and complete the task of mourning. We will then, once again, be able to gather the fruits of life. This mentally retarded child offers us a wisdom that reaches deeper than our reason can penetrate. Mourning seems wasteful and meaningless according to strict logic. Why grieve for something irretrievably lost? It makes no sense. Yet a wiser voice also speaks through us. It says: "Rage and protest, cry out in anguish and then the raw wounds will heal." There is a general progression of feeling states that usually make up the work of mourning. Although the intensity of each phase varies with the importance of the loss, the progression of feelings is often quite similar. And, as we have seen, grief is proportional to the reflected meaning of what has been lost.

The general emotional phases of mourning have been portrayed by many writers.[14] For the most part, all agree on three primary stages: the period of *shock and disbelief,* the period of *emerging awareness and intense emotion* and the period of *resolution.* * Every person will experience each stage differently, while some of us will experi-

---

*The stages of dying described by Kübler-Ross[15] are often oversimplified and misunderstood. They were never intended as a rigid guide and do not apply to only the experience of dying. They do, however, provide a conceptual framework within which each of us can deepen our understanding of loss. Every important loss has the inherent potential for carrying us through the Kübler-Ross phases of Denial, Anger, Bargaining, Depression and Acceptance. These are beautifully portrayed in her book *On Death and Dying.* Each emotional phase is contained within the stages we will discuss but more explicitly and with many more examples. Knapp and Hansen[16] have also shown that the parents of children with leukemia frequently experience the same sequential stages: the initial refusal to accept the diagnosis; the rage at God, the physician, hospital personnel, family members or the sick child when the reality of cancer can no longer be denied; participation in helpful activities to bargain for more time; grief when it becomes undeniably apparent that the child will die and finally acceptance of the inevitable death.

ence chaotic waves of feeling that could never have been anticipated
or neatly categorized. Yet we are all human and our differences do
not exceed the boundaries of our humanness. An understanding of
the general phases of human response can therefore act as a reference: as an imperfect map of an uncharted continent compounded
from reports of explorers who have gone before us and who spoke
of mountains in one region, forbidding storms in another and tran-
quil valleys near journey's end. Each of us takes a different and
unique pathway. And each of us can come to know that he is not
alone or lost in an uninhabited wilderness. We can learn of the
mountains, storms and valleys that we might encounter and know
that we will be neither the first nor the last to be so confronted. I
believe these stages can provide a frame of reference with which to
compare the uniqueness of one's experiences.

We must, however, understand that all such maps may become an
oppressive and doctrinaire system when they are misused. If viewed
as the "correct" sequence or the "right way" to experience loss, they
become a tyrannical invasion of privacy and strip the intimidated
patient of uniqueness and human integrity. There is no right way or
proper sequence. There are only heart and intelligence, courage and
our human spirit. It is with this perspective that I present the following general phases of mourning.

Shock and Disbelief. The feelings might be stated thus: "It isn't
possible, it can't be true; I can't have a malignancy, my physical
wholeness cannot be irretrievably lost, this loved person cannot be
irrevocably dead." Everything seems to be in a suspended state, like
a cartoon character who has run over the edge of a cliff and remains
momentarily poised in space, groping for lost ground, slowly becoming aware that there is only air beneath him. In the midst of such
shock, we might collapse into a paralyzed numbness, yearn for solitude, fly into a flurry of activities, try to stay a step ahead of denied
reality. Suggestions are irrelevant at best and are often experienced
by the mourner as irritating. Sympathetic condolence offered to a
mourner who is trying to ignore reality can be equally unsettling.
Mourners are trying to build an emotional equilibrium that will

allow them to accept the loss sustained. In such circumstances, some of us intellectually comprehend all the realities and behave in a perfectly appropriate manner, but the shock and disbelief are below the surface and tightly sealed off from awareness.

The period of shock and disbelief is usually experienced with incomprehension. It is one of those overwhelming moments in which no theory or counsel can help. It is only possible to cling to the knowledge that all aspects of grief are natural, including irrational thoughts and extreme behavior. There is no way to minimize shock and disbelief, but there are attitudes of acceptance which may prevent shame and bewilderment from joining it.

Despite the means of temporary protection utilized, the dreadful reality begins to seep through our emotional barricades with intermittent flashes of perception. Within hours or days, each of us begins to lower the walls of disbelief and admit as much despair as can be tolerated. Except in rare instances, shock and disbelief will quite naturally fade into the next phase of mourning. It is extremely ill advised for anyone to impose his individual behavior prescriptions on others. The process of transition is so personal that the mourner is truly the only expert on his own needs and feelings.

Emerging Awareness. As the reality of loss emerges into awareness, temporary numbness and flights into distracting activity begin to subside. Emptiness, despair and outrage are then the most prominent experiences of mourning. There is a violent need to cry out, to weep, to rage at anyone held responsible for the loss, to be a child in distress. This need is present whether a culture encourages public lamentation or a stiff upper lip. Regressing back to a childlike state can be a frightening and disturbing experience. Irrational behavior and intense emotion are often perceived with shame and revulsion, and there can be the accompanying fear that this childlike emotional state will last forever. But all of these surging feelings are an important part of the work of mourning.

There is often a compulsion to seek out the dead person during this period of intense grief. Signs of his or her presence are desperately needed. Hearing a voice or seeking out a spiritualist are com-

mon means of trying to bring back the loved one. Many people also
search through dream after dream. A young woman with whom I
once worked was given a pet squirrel by her husband. The squirrel
died shortly before he was killed and the two became fused in her
mind. She spent countless hours seeking her husband in the woods
and parks they had known together. She understood that she was
behaving irrationally but still hoped to find his spirit among the
squirrels she pursued. Most of us do not embark on such explicit
quests. We more commonly experience a distracted inattentiveness
with everything other than the deceased. These desperate searches
subside, they contain less of the supernatural, and they finally become transformed into cherished memories as the reality of loss
becomes integrated.

Intense weeping, the primary emotion of grief, is both a release
and a means of contact with others. There can be no lonelier time
in one's life than these dark and sad hours. It is therefore a great
comfort to be able to share grief with another person. To accept
one's grief is a personal achievement for it reflects great self-respect.
Expressions of extreme fear, anger and hostility, dramatically different from the mourner's normal personality, can burst forth. The
anger can be directed at the medical profession, at friends and family
and *at the dead person.* The fear and the hostility grow out of the pain
of abandonment. Survivors attack both those who failed to save the
life and the deceased themselves for having died and inflicted such
painful deprivation. Hate and love become fused. This ambivalence
is common and seen most dramatically in a child who has lost a
parent. The child's despair is rivaled by the murderous rage at being
abandoned. Since children cannot separate thought from consequence and usually assume full responsibility for everything that
happens, it is easy for them to believe retrospectively that their rage
drove the parent away. This self-centered omnipotence is partially
revived in every adult mourner who has had ambivalent feelings
about the deceased. Intense grief can start with guilt and self-
reproach and move on to the more direct and uncontaminated experience of loss.

We know that the intense experience of grief attends the loss of anything highly valued or anyone deeply loved. It is anticipated. But it is confusing for family members to experience the same deep sadness for a disliked parent or spouse or for a seemingly unimportant parent or spouse. The confusion results from the surprising disparity between importance of loss and depth of feeling. One man, puzzled by his strong grief following the death of his father, said: "I never got a thing from my old man. I didn't think I'd give a damn. I haven't even seen him for years, haven't wanted to. So I don't know what's getting to me."[17] One woman said: "David was a cold and unpleasant man to live with. I was so relieved to get divorced and get away from him. We talked a little during the last four or five years but he has been out of my life for a long time. Then I heard he had cancer and I felt so sad. I just don't know why, but, see what's happening, I start crying when I think of him."[18]

In some instances, these feelings of grief are expressions of childhood. They are the experiences of the child who still resides within the adult mourner. They reflect how that child would have felt if he had lost his mommy or daddy. The grief of the adult may arise from a time when there was no one else for the child to turn to.

In other instances, the unexpected feelings of sadness reveal a tenacious hope. When any of us yearn for love, recognition and acceptance, associate the longing with a specific person and are then frustrated for a period of years, it is common to hope that the person will one day fulfill our expectation, that he will finally see and love us. It might be obvious that the longed-for response will never happen, there might be overwhelming evidence that this persistent yearning is futile, but the hope still persists. It can be maintained by need and longing for as long as the person remains physically alive. Death or serious illness is then experienced as the undeniable final loss of this tenacious hope. The depth of grief does not represent the actual importance of the person but rather reflects the strength of the yearning for a love never given, a recognition never bestowed and an acceptance never offered. When death occurs, the process of mourning a reawakened childhood loss or the last vestiges of a persistent hopeful yearning can be as difficult and as painful as any experience of grief.

The often-quoted cliché remains absolutely true; each of us must try to remain true to himself. If this means disregarding authoritative advice which urges us to be strong and not to surrender to the pain of bereavement, we must disregard this inappropriate advice. If this means mourning in solitude, much as a wild animal might withdraw into the forest to heal its wounds, we must resist the pressure to grieve publicly. If this means refusing to shed insincere tears, we must examine this refusal and honor its truth. All expressions of grief should be respected. All styles and patterns and rhythms are valid. The greater the love and the stronger the emotional bond between one person and another, the more difficult and painful will be the mourning, the less graceful will be the letting go. As one woman said: "If no man's life were significant enough to cause weeping, if birth and death were unmarked, if the measure of our years on earth were nothing, we might better be houseflies rather than human beings."[19]

Resolution. Mourning, like any natural process, resolves itself when unobstructed. There are, however, several means of facilitating the process of mourning. Cultural rituals such as funeral services and family gatherings can serve to acknowledge the reality of death in a socially supportive setting. These public acknowledgments help to bring awareness and a sense of ending to the physical life of the deceased. The desire to visit the cemetery should not be discouraged, especially with children, for it is an excellent way to experience the painful finality of physical death and thereby foster the work of mourning. It is a shame that loss other than death cannot be ritualized and made more concrete. Religious beliefs can also bring comfort to the individual and aid the process of mourning.

As the months go by, the preoccupation and the intense sadness lessen, the memories evoke less guilt and ambivalence, and the mourner takes his or her place in the continuing pattern of life. More often than not, mourners at first feel more comfortable with other mourners, more open and empathetic, closer through shared loss. With time, there is a reawakened interest in other people and other things not directly related to loss and grief.

The pace at which resolution takes place often depends on prior attitudes toward potential loss. We can all engage in *preparatory mourning.* In this process we force ourselves to consider the idea of death and potential loss. By becoming familiar with these emotions and with their personal ramifications, we can learn to be more open and accepting of them. When death and loss seem likely, there is the more immediate process of *anticipatory mourning,* in which an actual person's death is mourned while he is alive. When a family grieves openly prior to death there is often less anguish following it. It is quite common for a family to draw close, grieve together and share their sadness. When this happens, the work of mourning will be greatly enhanced and the support so derived is immeasurable. It is well established that when there is no anticipatory grief, as with sudden deaths, the work of mourning is harder and longer and more complex.[20] The process of mourning will always be fostered by anticipating and experiencing grief in advance.

There are, however, some of us who become "stuck" and cannot proceed with the process of mourning. A child who has lost a parent or close sibling is especially prone to this problem. In such instances, a brief psycho-therapeutic experience can be enormously helpful and should be encouraged.

When Mourning Is Complete. The emotional pain caused by loss suffered does not move toward forgetfulness. It moves, rather, in the direction of enriched remembrance; the memory becomes an integral part of the mourner's personality. The work of mourning has been completed when the person (or cherished thing) no longer appears as an absence in a barren world but has come to reside securely within one's heart. Each of us must grieve in his own manner and at his own pace. For many people, one year seems to bring completion. Others require much more or much less time. Periodic waves of grief are often felt for the remainder of one's life. The mourning process must be given the freedom to find its own depth and rhythm; it cannot be artificially accelerated. A loss, like a physical wound, cannot heal overnight. There is no way to hurry the stages of tissue growth and there is no way to speed up the healing process of mourning. But, when mourning has been completed, the mourner comes to feel the inner presence of the loved one, no longer an idealized hero or a maligned villain, but a presence with human dimensions. Lost irreversibly in objective time, the person is present in a new form within one's mind and heart, tenderly present in inner time without the pain and bitterness of death. And once the loved one has been accepted in this way he can never again be forcefully removed.

My father died over ten years ago. He was the most important and deeply loved person in my life. I partially grieved his death but could gain no sense of completion and built a wall around my sadness. Six months after he died I had a dream. It remains as vivid today as it did the night it occurred. This is the dream:

Dad has been permitted to come back for one evening to bid us farewell. My mother, sister and I are having dinner with him. The conversation is lively, filled with teasing and good humor. It is my father who keeps the talk away from what we all know—that he is with us for a short and final visit. I become more and more sad as we laugh and talk but acquiesce to his happy banter. As it grows dark, we all lie down, my father and mother in their bed, my sister and I in a smaller one next to theirs. A night table stands between the beds, between my father and me. No one speaks, time passes, my sister and mother fall asleep, my dad and I lie quietly in the dark a few feet apart. I know that he is afraid to say anything, afraid that he might disturb or cause me pain. I want to reach out but am intimidated by the sacredness of his visit from the dead. A long time passes. Finally he reaches out his arm and places his open hand upon the table. I begin to tremble. This is so much like him. I can take his hand if I wish or decline his offer. I know there will be no reproach if I refuse. He waits patiently for me to decide. I slowly reach out and grasp his hand. When he feels my hand in his, he laughs tenderly, swings around and beams at me. We sit smiling at one another and then embrace for a long moment and then I am awake, alone and weeping.

To this day, it is hard for me to believe that the visit was only a dream. No waking experience has ever been more vivid. I needed to say goodbye and grieve his death, the visit occurred, the loving farewell was enacted and the work of mourning proceeded. If we are open to our grief, we will each find a path through the despair that surrounds us and we will each repossess within our hearts that which has been lost from the external world.

There is one last and important point I wish to make concerning the work of mourning. The process should come to an end. There is a strong likelihood that grief is being unintentionally exploited if it continues for many years. Endless mourning can be used as a means of refusing to accept life without the lost person. The mourner, in effect, is saying: "If I can't have things the way I want them to be, I won't participate in life at all." The avoidance of personal responsibility, the insistence on remaining forever in a helpless dependent situation, and at times the frozen and inflated idealization of a loved one can block the road back to people, work and a meaningful engagement with life. This stubborn refusal is self-imposed, often romanticized, and is, in truth, a form of partial suicide. The task is not to try harder to forget the loved one, since that effort only intensifies the mourner's total absorption with the deceased. The task is rather to direct one's attention elsewhere, to begin to do things and to see other people. The difficult part of these activities is the sense of meaninglessness in the effort, the sense of just going through the motions. Some people even feel a sense of betrayal, as if the past demands an eternal faithfulness. But the efforts are an affirmation of life and offer hope of reemergence. Probably the last and most subtle part of the work of mourning is that final letting go of a secret hope, the poignant wish that the loss had never occurred.

PART TWO

The Sphere of Personal Influence

The diagnosis and treatment of cancer are often experienced as an assault upon our sense of well-being. The circumstances of our lives, the bodies we inhabit, the very thoughts and emotions that define our sense of self seem on the verge of raging out of control. And yet the great majority of us do not fall apart. We reestablish our sense of equilibrium and continue our lives. The turbulent anxieties, depressions, rages and frustrations subside. We adjust to new circumstances and, in many instances, grow richer in wisdom and self-respect.

But how does one approach the pain and confusion of the cancer crisis? How are these formidable tasks accomplished? What are the processes of restoration and growth? There are literally dozens of coping strategies commonly used during times of stress. Some of us turn toward outside sources of help; we derive emotional support from loved ones, seek out those who have experienced similar circumstances, search for new and sustaining activities. Some of us instinctively turn toward our ability to reason and analyze; we separate the probable from the unlikely, cause from effect; we focus our attention, clarify our thoughts, modify our expectations and anticipate the consequences of various possible behaviors. Some try to turn away from distress. Others hope to find a guiding principle or a means of fulfillment within it. This section will explore that sphere in which each of us can exert a significant personal influence on the events and experiences of the cancer crisis.

4

The Politics of Integrity

It pleases me and seems right that what is of value and
wisdom to one man seems nonsense to another.
—HERMANN HESSE

Each of us has a characteristic way of responding to events, be they
external realities such as the diagnosis and treatment of cancer, or
internal realities such as the intense emotions evoked by such events.
There is no sudden shift in our personality during the stress of cancer
treatment. Rather there is an increasing consistency: long-standing
values become dearer, childhood experiences become more vivid
and lingering fears become more ominous. Individual perceptions
and experiences are realities in themselves and can dominate the life
quality of the cancer crisis as readily as surgery or radiation therapy.

Two Kinds of Parents

Imagine a child attempting something new, something difficult
and frightening. Now imagine a parent: one who supports and respects the child, who calls for a genuine effort and offers firm,
consistent support, feeling both pride in the child's progress and
sympathy during inevitable failures. Now imagine another parent
guiding the same child's attempts at a difficult task, a parent who

demands immediate success, who is impatient and tolerates no mistakes, who is harsh and punitive and perfectionistic. There is no doubt which parent is the more likely to foster self-confidence and self-esteem. Yet when we ourselves approach something new and frightening, when a small part in each of us once again resembles a child struggling to succeed, we all too often become a harsh, vindictive, abusive parent to that struggling part of ourselves. We condemn, berate, undermine and vilify; we take no measure of pride in tasks completed and permit ourselves to feel no pleasure in progress we have made. We see only defects and deficiencies. Some of us even manage to condemn ourselves for being self-condemning, and in doing so choose to engage in precisely that kind of endless accusation guaranteed to wound the childlike part of every adult under stress. I believe wholeheartedly that we are all capable of adopting the attitude of a firm, empathetic and understanding parent toward this frightened and aspiring aspect of ourselves and others. I ask you to share this bias toward greater self-acceptance and to approach these issues of adjustment in a spirit of empathetic curiosity, with the courage of a kind parent.

Every adaptive strategy has both advantages and disadvantages. Knowledge of them permits a far greater range of choice and effectiveness. We would therefore do well to establish a framework of reference within which to consider these various approaches and potential behaviors. We would also do well to have a rough sense of temperamental differences, a sense of those strategies which tend to satisfy different temperamental needs.

Zelda and Miriam

Having considered two divergent *parental attitudes,* let us now consider two children who bring vastly different temperaments to the experience of facing something that is unknown. Robert W. White[1] discusses two three-year-old children on their first visit to a school psychologist. The experience of being tested by a strange woman may seem simple enough to us, but it is a major and frightening undertaking for most three-year-olds. It is possible to learn a great deal about ourselves and particularly about our responses to stress by observing the way in which these two children go about their task of facing a frightening encounter. I will refer to the first young lady as Zelda, the second as Miriam.[2]

Zelda enters the testing room without hesitation, performs each of the test requirements, seems interested, charms everyone with her friendly smile, makes conversation, asks for help when she needs it and thanks the psychologist at the end of the session. Miriam comes in reluctantly and says nothing. She stands beside her mother and won't sit down. She finally begins to string beads only after her mother has done so first. Once she is familiar and proficient with them, she is reluctant to perform the other activities suggested by the psychologist, now eager to continue the test. Miriam does eventually comply but the testing is erratic because she keeps getting involved with little projects of her own design rather than those requested by the psychologist. The test is only half completed when the session is over.

What conclusions might be drawn about these two youngsters? A typical assessment would describe Zelda as mature, confident, independent and remarkably well adjusted. Miriam would not fare so well. She might be criticized for clinging to her mother and for not cooperating with the "nice lady." Her assessment might read: suffers from separation anxiety and refuses to respond appropriately to social stimulation. But a great deal that is relevant to our discussion is not reflected in such convenient assessment. Prior to their session, neither Zelda nor Miriam knows who this strange psychologist is or what she will do to them. They are each being asked to participate in something new and they cannot help but be a little frightened. It seems, from a child's perspective, that Zelda is expecting the testing to be as much fun as mom has promised, that she has convinced herself there is really nothing to fear. Zelda therefore steps easily into the unknown circumstance; her strategy is one of reliance and trust. Miriam is not nearly so sure of what might be in store for her, and her behavior accomplishes three fundamental tasks during the testing session: she seeks information, digests it at her own pace and diligently maintains her personal autonomy. Upon entering the psychologist's office, she stays close to mom, her one familiar object. She uses this secure "home base" to survey the room and gather up information. She consents to participate in only those activities she understands. Her delays and refusals, although frustrating for the psychologist, allow her to maintain her equilibrium and give her time to digest these new perceptions and experiences.

If we compare the strategies of Miriam with those of Zelda, we find that each approach has advantages and disadvantages. Miriam, even at the age of three, derives the benefit of being her own person and respecting her own private needs. But she must suffer disapproval and unpopularity. Zelda is admired, approved of and adored. She has obviously developed a robust ability to trust herself and others. But her world will not always remain safe and protected. Zelda will surely experience a stinging bewilderment when her indiscriminate trust encounters the indifference and competitiveness of adolescence. Fate can indeed bring cruel blows and bitter disappointment. Without further development of her adaptive skills, she will experience a growing vulnerability, for she will have exchanged her personal authority and emerging competence for the comforting belief that others will always be kind and capable.

Zelda, Miriam and the Cancer Crisis. Zelda and Miriam represent two distinct prototypes of behavior, two distinct temperamental attitudes toward stress. Each child will mature in her own way. Zelda will probably acquire many new adaptive skills as she navigates her way through childhood and young adulthood. Miriam will no doubt overcome her timidness and develop a greater trust in others. But as adults, during the cancer crisis, Zelda and Miriam will often revert to these childhood strategies. Zelda will tend to *rely* on her ability to believe in others. Miriam will tend to utilize her ability to assess information, understand consequences, make her own independent decisions and maintain her *autonomy*. Each of us, when confronted by the demands and stresses of the cancer crisis, tends to seek our own adaptive style. This response usually contains a mixture of Zelda "reliance" and Miriam "autonomy" and it is not difficult to recognize the adult forms of each tendency in ourselves and in others.

A diagnosis of malignancy is made; dreadful images are evoked and they are hard to dispel; major treatment is suggested by a stranger who, we are told, is a competent specialist. How is one to proceed? Those of us who share personality traits with Zelda seek out a trustworthy physician and place ourselves in this expert's capable hands. We try to be good patients, follow instructions and make minimal demands. In doing so, we are praised as the ideal patients, the agreeable family members, and are the joy of every doctor or hospital ward. This *reliant* style has many advantages. Establishing a relationship with a skilled and competent cancer specialist allows us to believe that "the doctor knows best"; it permits us to place everything in his experienced hands. The benefits of such confidence are immediately apparent. Anxiety is reduced and control is usually reestablished when a knowledgeable, kind, parental authority assumes total responsibility for the stressful problem. While under this protective umbrella, one can experience a great deal of reassurance. These are distinct advantages. Being able to trust those upon whom we must depend is essential since all of us entering cancer treatment must submit to medical intervention. But there are also problems. A sense of control and safety has been achieved, in large part, through the urgent delegation of responsibility. Having gambled on the goodness of others, having declined to participate actively in the hard decisions of treatment, having only searched for a protective refuge, the patient is in a vulnerable and precariously dependent state. If mistrust, doubt, disapproval or failure becomes associated with the patient's "protector," a great deal of anxiety can attend the *reliant* strategy of adaptation. Fear of abandonment and feelings of helplessness accompany the loss or the threatened loss of this protected refuge. Those of us who resemble adult versions of Zelda are emotional gamblers. We seek out the best in others and attach our hopes to their abilities. We also often disregard our own capacity to influence the events of our lives.

Those of us who share personality traits with Miriam proceed quite differently: we search for some means of remaining in charge of ourselves. Our anxiety escalates under conditions of imposed dependency. We do much better when able to participate in the treatment process. We might need to go to the hospital alone or to delay certain treatment procedures until we are emotionally prepared. We need to be informed and to be included in all important decisions. Those of us with the *autonomous* strategy of adaptation experience a reduction of anxiety by retaining a sense of personal authority and by not letting go of our independent status. There are advantages and disadvantages to this approach as well. Although personal authority and competence can be maintained, those with tendencies toward autonomy are often disliked and criticized by health professionals. They are often made to feel like uncooperative, pig-headed, ungrateful irritants who upset clinic routines. Patients and family members are therefore afraid of retaliations. Inner turmoil can be even more destructive to more autonomous patients and family members than the experience of being disliked. Doubt and anxiety accompany most attempts to assume responsibility, and the ensuing inner conflicts can become extremely painful.

Adaptation as Process. *Reliant* and *autonomous* patients control their degree of awareness, both seek a safe emotional stability and both yearn for the presence of a strong and competent authority. But they approach these goals quite differently. *Reliant* patients achieve an emotional stability by controlling information and remaining unaware of those things that evoke anxiety. They maintain a feeling of safety through the delegation of responsibility and authority. *Autonomous* patients try to be as aware as possible, and they attempt to establish a state of inner stability by integrating the realities with which they are confronted. Most importantly, they attempt to maintain this stability through the assertion of personal authority. Each of us, regardless of his own unique mixture of reliance and autonomy, is trying to reduce anxiety and to regain a sense of lost control. There are times in which the best of all possible adjustments must include loss, suffering and bitter frustration. Adapting oneself to an altered body or a changed environment often requires the acceptance of disheartening conditions. It is therefore important to understand that there is no "end product" or "final solution." A well-adjusted person is someone who deals with these enormous demands in a self-accepting and relatively productive manner.

The management of the cancer crisis is a *process* of adaptation. There are a variety of attitudes and approaches. Each can be appropriate and we must try to give ourselves permission to utilize any adaptive strategy that seems promising. Every approach is a part of a process that contains implicit tasks. These include: (1) the acquisition of information at a pace that allays anxiety; (2) the establishment of sufficient emotional stability to deal with the stress; and (for the autonomous) (3) the maintenance of a sense of personal authority. We will explore these three tasks. The first, controlling one's level of awareness and monitoring information, is an important part of the process of adaptation and an extremely controversial subject. Physicians and family members ponder the question of telling the patient the "whole truth"; patients (and at times family members) struggle with the dilemma of how much they want to know. Important decisions cannot be made with insufficient knowledge nor can they be made in the state of emotional chaos which may be caused by receiving too much information too quickly. Neither extreme allows the establishment of the kind of emotional stability that makes it possible to integrate changing realities and to make appropriate choices. There are clear principles to be discovered about these questions of telling, about these conflicting wishes to know and not know, and they are all related to questions of personal integrity.

To Know and to Know Not

All of us approach the unknown differently. But once the diagnosis of cancer has been made, once the process of treatment has begun, everyone, regardless of temperamental preference, must also face the attitudes imposed upon him by hospital administrators and physicians. There are therefore two determining factors: our own attitudes and those attitudes to which we are subjected. Unfortunately, internal and external attitudes often reflect divergent needs, and this discordance results in additional stress. Although there has been a great deal of recent interest in and a greatly expanded sensitivity to the human side of cancer, questions of "telling the whole truth" are still as controversial and painful as ever. Most doctors (88 percent in one study) elect not to tell the truth even when patients ask if they have cancer.[3] This pervasive attitude seems remarkable in light of the fact that almost all cancer patients are quite aware of their diagnosis.[4] It is not surprising that most cancer patients know that they have cancer. In fact, it seems unlikely that many people could go through such highly specialized diagnostic procedures as mammography, cytology and biopsy, followed by recommendations for surgery or radiation therapy, without having some awareness that the disease being investigated and treated is cancer. And in advanced stages the terrible truth that no curative treatment is available and that the patient will die cannot be hidden from anyone who does not choose to deceive themself. Doctors, friends and especially family members are extremely poor actors. Symptoms persist and excuses are unconvincing. Most experts agree that "a patient who is sick enough to die knows it without being told."[5]

This awareness applies to children as well. Adults might deceive themselves into believing that children suspect nothing, but they rarely deceive a child over the age of three.[6] Isolating a child who is confused and afraid is neither protective nor kind. Children quickly become aware that something is seriously wrong. If we put ourselves in a child's shoes for a moment we can easily imagine the tone of conversations overheard, the furtive looks observed, the sound of false reassurance, the grim hospital procedures, even the special attention received. Ominous hints are everywhere and every large-eyed child is alert to these blatant cues. They might worry in silence. But they worry. Concern is expressed in their faces, in their careful questions, in their dreams and even in their jokes.

Laurie was ten years old and had leukemia. As time went by she became increasingly sullen and refused to take medicine or follow her parents' instructions. No one could understand why she was so disagreeable. There was, however, no mystery about her behavior. She was furious at her parents for what she experienced to be their lack of concern. They did not want her to worry and therefore behaved in a cheerful and evasive manner. But she felt abandoned and outraged by this emotional desertion. Laurie's angry behavior stopped the moment they began to be open and honest.[7]

And yet most physicians and many families arbitrarily choose not to comment on the presence of cancer, on a fact well known to most patients. When this happens, everyone is caught in the game of "let's pretend." As one experienced nurse states: "The staff think they are sparing the patient untold misery by pretending, while the patient thinks he is sparing the staff endless discomfort by playing along. And so it goes for weeks and months."[8]

There are many reasons offered by cancer specialists for not being honest about the diagnosis of cancer. Among the most frequently cited are: the truth will upset the patient and cause depression or actual physical deterioration; patients don't really want to know; patients are harder to manage when they know, for the truth makes them so agitated that they run off to cancer quacks; it is more stressful for the family when the patient knows; knowing increases the risk of suicide.[9] The justification that underlies each reason could be stated thus: "It is really kinder not to tell." However, it is usually the condition of ignorance that causes stress. The contorted efforts at concealment and strained reassurance which must follow the original lie cannot help but create mistrust and bitterness in everyone involved. In fact, deceit and ignorance, even though well intentioned, can become a force that greatly magnifies anxiety and depression. Suicide is extremely rare among cancer patients and studies have shown that nearly 90 percent of all cancer patients say they want to be told the truth.[10] As far as kindness is concerned, it is necessary to ask the embarrassing question: kinder for whom? Kinder for the person who must do the telling, kinder for the family member who must openly share the pain of this monumental reality?

The Principle of Patient Guidance

A principle begins to emerge from these observations: since cancer patients are the only people who truly know what is best for them, they must become the experts who guide the process of adaptation and determine the amount of information they require. Those of us who tend toward a *reliant* style of adaptation will be comforted by management that is remarkably different from that requested by those of us who tend toward an *autonomous* style. But regardless of temperamental preference the same principle holds true: patients must determine their own mode of acquiring stressful information.

Since most cancer patients know that they have cancer (or that something is terribly wrong), the raging debate over whether or not to tell the truth is irrelevant. The essential struggle resides within every cancer patient and concerns *how much* they want to know. Stated more precisely, it concerns how much information and how much awareness they will permit themselves to have at any one moment. The emotional subtleties of this universal human conflict can be known only by the one who experiences it. The imposition upon the patient of personal theories and assumptions can be both irrelevant and grossly misguided.

Those of us who are comforted by the delegation of responsibility to others (the more reliant) might never want to hear or assimilate the fact of cancer, and we have ways to let this preference be known. We can change the subject whenever the diagnosis is referred to or insist that "it is only an infection." We can forget or reinterpret what has been said. One such patient, told that he had a malignant tumor, was later asked what he believed it to be. He replied: "A condition which, if you don't take care of yourself, will develop into cancer." He also said: "If I actually got cancer, I'm afraid I'd go crazy."[11] Some patients instruct us very explicitly. One doctor told his patient that he had read the pathologist's report and knew the test results; the patient, however, replied forcibly: "Well, I don't!" The doctor said: "You mean you don't want me to tell you?" The patient again replied emphatically: "That's right!"[11] Another simply said: "If it's something bad, don't tell me."[12]

These patients are guiding their physicians and family members with direct and clearly stated instructions. They are taking care of their needs in an admirable and self-respecting manner. They are asserting their right to protect a vitally needed emotional equilibrium and are instructing the "senders" of potentially distressful information as to how they can help them most at that particular moment. Patients with this extreme approach are most comforted by assuming the role of sick children and are hoping to be cared for by knowledgeable, helpful and responsible adults. They have a need to be relatively unaware of what is happening and gain reassurance through the act of placing themselves in the capable hands of others. Such extreme responses are not rare and are a valid emotional strategy.

The other extreme, of complete autonomy, is also common and can be easily illustrated by such statements as: "I want to know everything and I mean everything"; "My worst fear is that I'll be kept in the dark"; "It's my life, how dare they try to steal it?" [*How are they doing that?*] "By not telling me exactly what's happening."[13] The bitter experience of a librarian exemplifies this need to acquire *all* relevant information. After being told by a specialist that she had a malignant tumor of the cervix and that it required surgery, the patient, as a good solid New Englander, showed little emotion. "She made a date for surgery and walked out of the office to think it over. She then proceeded to the library, methodically took out all the latest journals in the field and began reading the statistics as well as the preferred surgical procedures. She called her physician in order to make an appointment to discuss the details and the management of her case. He was quite blunt and asked her to leave these matters in his hands. She felt rebuffed and canceled the surgery. She insisted that while the surgeon might be an outstanding technician, he could not be her doctor because he didn't know how to deal with her kind of person."[14] And she was right! The surgeon she had consulted treated all his patients as if they possessed the same temperamental needs. Had he asked someone with a *reliant* temperament to "leave these matters in my hands," he would have been offering the most comforting assurance possible. But the temperament of this fiercely independent librarian was intensely autonomous, and therefore the authoritarian imposition of the doctor's absolute power evoked anxiety and drove her away.

Most of our responses and temperamental requirements lie between these two extremes. Most of us possess varied and shifting

needs; we seek information at one moment and recede from awareness at another. Although the signals we send might be considerably
more subtle than those quoted above, although our desires might be
considerably more ambivalent, the principle of "patient guidance"
remains absolutely valid. Those of us who elect to resist emerging
awareness hope for an inner stability based on "protected innocence." Those of us who strive to maintain a feeling of personal
authority and competence hope to achieve an inner stability through
the integrated awareness of what is happening to us. Let us consider
this latter need for precise and explicit information.

Facts and Catastrophic Fantasies

We all have unique mechanisms for dealing with painful realities.
But, without information, without realities to deal with, most of us
are likely to contrive "fantasy facts" in an effort to explain events.
What we conjure up to fill in the empty spaces left by insufficient
information can be far more frightening than the painful realities
themselves.

Fear of flying is a common experience and a dramatic metaphor.
A great many people are particularly distressed in an airplane by the
feeling of being in danger and out of control. Severe anxiety
emerges from the dreadful fantasies associated with the ungrounded
experience of being carried away by a powerful force. However,
many people are reassured when they know exactly what is happening to them. World heavyweight boxing champion Muhammad Ali,
known for his courage and willingness to face great challenges, had
a lifelong terror of flying and refused to fly for many years. He once
said: "I don't like airplanes. But I think if I was in one, right beside
the pilot, and he show me how the motor works, explain things to
me about turbulence, and I could run the motor on the ground a
while and listen to it, then I'd feel safe. If he could tell me, if a motor
conked out, how far we could glide . . ."[15]. Ali was searching for
a way to remain in control and required precise information. Knowing exactly what the plane and pilot are really like makes it possible

for him to replace a terrifying fantasy with newly discovered facts and to establish a comprehensible world of reality. Knowledge of this kind works. Ali has been flying around the world now for many years.

All of us are capable of reducing the extreme anxiety associated with cancer treatment by replacing fantasies created out of fear and ignorance with the unpleasant but concrete realities of actual treatment. One way of treating children who are plagued with recurrent nightmares is to have them draw or paint their nocturnal monsters in as much horrifying detail as possible. When brought out of the dark of night and into the safe light of day, most children begin to ridicule the terrible monsters and then find it possible to minimize their fear. The secret is simple. As dark and ominous fantasies, the nightmare monsters are overwhelming; as concrete images seen in daylight, they become manageable. The same holds true for the terrifying fantasies that accompany the diagnosis and treatment of cancer. Information, understanding and the courage to confront the unknown make it possible to bring the nightmare images of cancer into the light of day. The value of such "daytime" awareness cannot be overestimated. The *accuracy* of a patient's knowledge of treatment procedures has been shown to be highly correlated with levels of improvement during rehabilitation. The best-informed patients improve the most.[16]

Most of us have similar needs regarding the acquisition of medical information. We need answers when we want them and in language we can understand. We need some encouragement by the surgeon or radiation therapist to express our fears, for it is only by listening to these fantasies that a cancer expert can help us separate misconception from medical reality. We need an active sensitivity to our moods; both a vague response and an avalanche of unabsorbable information may be equally inappropriate and terrifying. A brief, permissive conversation, on the other hand, might well allow us to regain a sense of hope and competence.

There are enormous differences in our speed and capacity to process stressful information. We should never conclude that the most ready acceptance is necessarily the most adaptive or successful.

How well and how deeply such distressing knowledge has been integrated can only be known with time and experience. The fact that a patient feels considerable conflict and anxiety during the diagnostic workup does not necessarily mean that he is incapable of assimilating the fact of cancer. Even a vehement protest may be a healthy sign of eventual acceptance. Certainly each of us is hoping desperately that there is nothing seriously wrong while at the same time we are suspecting the worst. When we know what is happening, when we can become withdrawn, depressed, hysterical, when we are allowed to cry out in bitter outrage, *then* we can begin the slow process of integrating these realities and our responses to them. Only then might we call upon previously untapped personal resources or experience a profoundly new understanding of ourselves.

With knowledge, we can bring our strongest capabilities into an honest alliance with health professionals. In ignorance, most of us will no doubt suspect the worst, struggle with terrifying phantoms, begin to mistrust everyone and feel desperately alone.

Children need information in the same manner as adults. They can be distracted from their anxieties but will usually perceive the superficial dishonesty of this approach. The perception can lead to mistrust, fear, isolation and despair. A forthright manner, on the other hand, will result in an atmosphere of shared hope and in a reduction of the need for distraction. Even when one is facing death, knowing the truth (the fact of life-threatening illness) can resolve a great deal of stress. The father of a dying child, a physician himself, had to learn this lesson. "When my middle son was dying of certain incurable complications, I saw him become hostile and distrustful of everybody he loved best. It was making his final months dreadful for him and for us as well until I came to him and spelled out every last word of the truth. We cried together and from that time on he was close to us again and we to him."[17]

Parents of seriously ill children need to know what to expect: how their child might respond to medication or other treatment procedures, what physical and emotional symptoms might emerge and what they should do. Parents can help the treatment process enormously by understanding symptoms and by being aware of drug reactions and side effects. If they are denied participation, if they are subjected to the "idiot treatment," most seek information elsewhere and often misinform themselves. Family members have many important tasks to accomplish, and these require specific information. Simple, direct, honest answers are the best medicine that can be offered.

An Alternative to Protective Concealment

The only relevant issue is *how* information might best be shared. We must ask ourselves: "Is information being sought? Are subtle instructions being offered? If so, what are the messages and how can I honor them?" All of these questions are based on the basic principle that each patient should determine the manner in which stressful information is shared. This principle is infinitely preferable to the sweeping technique of protective concealment. If each patient clearly stated his current preference and each health professional (or family member) were sensitive and respectful of his needs, there would be a dramatic decrease in the stress of cancer treatment.

Most patients can be told the facts of their illness in a gentle and hopeful manner. In fact, most patients want and need to know. They have much to do and they require information in order to proceed with these tasks. Knowledge of a serious life-threatening illness will naturally produce shock, anxiety and depression. Once this information has been offered, the patient's needs must guide the process of information sharing. Questions should be answered truthfully by the physician, for the presentation of medical information is the physician's responsibility. Kind deceit is rarely justified. Garner's excellent guide offers a valuable step-by-step approach to the sharing of information concerning cancer treatment.[18] These steps consist of presenting the basic information (you have a tumor that requires surgery) in a hopeful context and discouraging the assumption that awareness can only bring disheartening information; respecting each patient's means of reducing anxiety and offering no more exact information than has been requested; telling the truth at all times but at a pace guided by the patient's questions; and offering an authentic encouragement based on the truth.

When realities are being denied, this denial should usually be accepted as a valuable protective device and not violated. The need to deny will usually diminish with time and lessened anxiety. But there are some of us who always maintain their "preference" for not knowing. Life goes on around this preference. Playwright Robert Anderson describes the four years during which his wife struggled with inoperable cancer: "To tell or not to tell? Why didn't I? Was it that I didn't trust her reaction or was it my reaction I didn't trust? Was it my war with reality? Five times we came to the point, 'I want to know what is happening to me.' Five times we made appointments with the doctor so that he could explain it to her completely. Five times she cancelled the appointment. She knew but she didn't want to know."[19]

It seems to me that Robert Anderson trusted her deeper needs and trusted himself in the most important way possible; he allowed her needs (no matter how varied or ambivalent) to guide his behavior; he allowed his wife to determine her own level of awareness. It was clearly the right choice, for she remained active during the greatest part of those years and did much of her major work as a writers' representative. This work resulted, at the time of her death, in eight books being dedicated to her, a theater named for her in New York and the establishment of scholarships and awards in her name at various universities. Paradoxically, she both knew and did not know the truth. "She wanted her favorite porcelain, Royal Copenhagen. We were told that there would be a two year delay. A quick look at me and she said, 'Oh, then there is no point.' I insisted there was a point. We had waited that long, we could wait another two years. She had enormous pleasure in choosing and ordering just what she wanted."[20] This woman knew that she was not going to live and chose not to directly acknowledge the fact to her husband or to herself. To have undermined her use of denial would have served no purpose; it would have been cruel and destructive. To think of her unique strategy of adaptation as "pathological" would also be absurd. She was a strong, gifted and independent woman who chose to remain unaware and succeeded at her own life task! There was never any reason to tell her more than she wanted to know.

All of us have the right and the need to monitor our own level of awareness. Most of us will choose to be more aware than Phyllis Anderson, but we all have the right to become aware of the precise amount of information we choose to handle. Open access and sensitive transfer of needed information are the responsibility of the physician and the family, while every patient is responsible for guiding the process of acquisition. It is an essential right and responsibility. And it is an important part of achieving the inner stability so necessary to deal with the cancer crisis.

5

Finding the Safe Place

I ask that you become a cave and shelter me, a large rock
behind which I can crouch, the hollow of a tree into
which I can squeeze myself, a hole in the earth made by
a blind creature who will not be frightened by my face.
—KIM CHERNIN, Unpublished Journal

The Need for Emotional Security

We would be perpetually on the raw edge of panic were it not
possible to reduce the disruptive force of anxiety following the
diagnosis of cancer. Controlling our level of awareness is one important way of reducing anxiety. There are *many* other ways as well, and
they range from primitive devices (simply not believing) to much
more sophisticated psychological strategies of protection. All approaches have the same basic goal: the establishment of greater
emotional safety. Mechanisms such as delay, avoidance, denial and
distortion are often described as major obstacles to cancer treatment.[1] However, the emotional protection and safety they offer can
be crucial to the patient.

The recognition and acknowledgment of symptoms suggesting
cancer can evoke a paralyzing dread. Going to a physician for an
examination can be experienced as rushing to one's execution.
Delay, like all adaptive strategies, is an important means of dealing
with potentially overwhelming anxiety even though it can reduce

the chances of cure. Although we must all try to confront behavior which obviously undermines life-saving treatment, the strategies by which we find greater emotional safety are adaptive and should command our respect. They help to maintain emotional integrity and prevent a terrifying descent into chaos. Every patient has the absolute right to determine his own degree of awareness, and we all must strive to respect this right.

Blatant denial of cancerlike symptoms requires our understanding. Being well informed about cancer, knowing the danger signals, having money and being familiar with community resources (all reasons to seek prompt consultation) *do not* reduce the tendency to deny and delay. Even people who are well aware of the fact that early detection greatly increases chances for cure tend to postpone. A physician says: "I had pain in my stomach off and on for the past several months, but you know how it is, I kept putting off going to see a doctor. I knew all the time what he'd find."[2] Knowledge and fear are not enough to offset these powerful protective mechanisms. It does no good to scold and scare and condemn. Those of us who have delayed are already frightened and guilty. We need an opportunity to confess and to be forgiven. We need acceptance much more than parental lectures. It took courage to come for an examination knowing that cancer might be diagnosed. The delay was understandable, not reprehensible, and there is every reason to experience a certain measure of pride in having overcome so much anxiety. Scolding is inappropriate, it serves no purpose, it can only burden the patient.

Here Is Your Place

All strategies of emotional protection are efforts to find a safe place, to create a reassuring and stable internal environment. That goal is beautifully expressed in the following account by a forty-year-old woman immersed in the cancer experience. "I've had a recurrent fantasy since the time I was thirteen. It always comes when I'm feeling scared, all alone and desperate. It comes when something terrible has just happened. I see it inside my head. The image and the voices are so clear that it's hard to believe they aren't real . . . for me they are. There are three hooded figures without faces, with a medieval quality. They stand before a slightly opened door with a little light peeking around its edges. As soon as I see them I begin to feel calm. They step aside, the door opens out very slowly and I begin to see a black universe with stars and a beautiful luminous green planet. Although I've never seen it completely, I can clearly make out that it is green and beautiful. It is a place for me, it is waiting for me. And then I hear a quiet voice say: 'Hold on, hold on and you'll have your place.' And at times it says: 'There is a purpose to all of this, here is your place and it's waiting for you.' Whenever this vision comes and the door opens and I hear the voice, I begin to feel at peace. No one can take it away from me, no one can steal the reassurance and comfort I feel. I hadn't seen the vision for many years but I always knew it was there if I really needed it. And it came last night. It would go away any time I wished. [*What might tempt you to send it away?*] It's a crutch . . . it's a little crazy, it's selfish to keep it just for myself. But I'll never give it up."[3]

I applaud this woman's ability to experience so beautiful and reassuring an image. The vision is an inherent part of her personality and an admirable means of dealing with stress and sorrow. It is a perfect symbol for all those strategies of adaptation which attempt to establish an inner quietness, a refuge from anxiety and doubt, a place of safe retreat.

The word *strategy* is derived from the name of the Greek general Strategos, who always had alternative plans in mind if his initial attempts were unsuccessful. Strategies designed to establish emotional stability may well fail. But, if they should, others are always available. Strategies may be open and obvious or they may be unknown even to the one who uses them. In many instances, we would prefer that they remain unknown. But the ability to accept ourselves and others during the cancer crisis often requires a knowledge of how the mind works and a sense of how many behaviors, which we discover with shame in ourselves, are, in fact, universal. What, then, are some of these strategies of adaptation and how do they work?

From among the many that offer a place of safety, we will examine the use of denial, regression, guilt and the illusion of omnipotence.

The Selective Denial of Reality

Many years ago, when my daughter was seven years old, I promised to take her to the San Francisco Zoo. The day of the trip arrived and so did an unexpected thunderstorm. She walked to the window, looked out through the downpour and said: "It's really not raining! Why can't we go?" She is an unusually intelligent and honest young lady, with perfect eyesight. But she, like all children and most adults, has the capacity to deny an unwelcome reality.

There are few circumstances that evoke a greater need to deny reality than the diagnosis and treatment of cancer. When such a reality does enter our lives, we yearn for a reprieve, for a time in which to prepare ourselves for the ordeal ahead. Temporary denial of what is happening to us is a common means of establishing the needed emotional protection. It can be used with the first symptom or with approaching death.

The greatest source of emotional stability and safety is hope. Panic subsides when there is hope of a cure. But, if treatment has failed to arrest tumor growth, a struggle between the awareness of approaching death and the denial of this awareness can emerge. It is common for a patient or a family member both to deny the reality of approaching death and at the same time to withdraw and mourn the imminent loss of life. The moods are contradictory and yet they complement one another; both serve the process of adapting to an inevitable reality. The denial provides a refuge and the grief fosters eventual acceptance. The same two complementary moods affect family members and friends. But questions arise. Should one support the hope expressed during periods of denial? Should one acknowledge the pessimism of despair? There are no easy answers and some people never resolve the conflict. They hold to their ambivalence even as they approach death.

Harold, one of our doctors, died of cancer several months ago. He worked here for seventeen years and was an unusually generous man. Everyone loved him. At one point he began to talk about his death and how he had come to accept it. It was Christmas time and he knew this was to be his last Christmas. But the next time we would talk, he was extolling the new spring and describing how he was going to fight to see another Christmas. And then later I'd see him once again accepting of death. Sometimes he would even switch in the middle of the same conversation. The nursing staff became agitated because he would not make up his mind and they never knew what to expect. I spent a lot of time with them talking about Harold's conflict and what it touched in each of us. We decided to try to accompany him through these extreme shifts and to try not to anticipate his moods. It became much easier for us and our increased comfort seemed to take a great deal of pressure off Harold. He never did choose. When he reached the final moments of his life, he held my hand and said: "I'll be okay." I never knew if he thought he would get well and was in that sense okay or if he had finally accepted his death.[4]

Harold's "okay" was undefined but it hardly matters which way he meant it. He had found a means of dealing with the anxiety and despair associated with his approaching death, while those who attended him discovered a way to respect and support his shifting needs. It is vitally important for all of us to understand that these emotional mood swings from hopeful denial to sad withdrawal are quite common. One woman, dying of cancer, never spoke of the possibility of death. She preferred to talk about her effective treatment and her plans to join the family at their summer home. Family, friends, doctors and nurses did not know that she was fully aware of her impending death. But a letter written long before she died contained expressions of devotion for her family and complete instructions for her funeral.[5]

The simple question "What can I do to help you right now?" will often provide specific information and guidance. Requests might include: the need for pain medication, the need to talk, the need to see a specific person, the need to perform a specific task, the need to be distracted, the need to be alone or the need to be of help to others. This simple question can remove a great deal of guesswork and false assumption. There are those who are immeasurably comforted by their capacity for denial and there are others who cannot keep their feelings and thoughts from swarming into awareness. Those who most benefit from denial prefer to become aware slowly and do so only in an atmosphere of warm support. Those with less ability to deny are uncomfortable in the presence of cautious tact and protective silence. They are more easily reassured by an honest "clearing of the air." An awareness of these temperamental differences may assist us in being more supportive and helpful. But the circumstances of denied reality usually remain confusing and may easily become frustrating for patient and family alike. We must all therefore struggle to respect its purpose and allow ourselves to be guided by the immediacy of each patient's needs.

Regression into Childhood

Once the reality of cancer is acknowledged, it becomes necessary to find a safe place within the ongoing process of cancer treatment. Many of us return to childlike behavior that once provided gratification. When an adult patient is in such a childlike state, he is basically saying: "All right, I'm seriously ill. Now someone else will have to take care of me." The behavior can range from sweet smiles to temper tantrums depending on temperament, but there is always a perceptibly childlike tone to it.

The regression to childhood is understandable. As a patient, each of us is removed from our familiar life and asked to be the passive recipient of "necessary" medical procedures. The confusion and dependency of such a state are characteristic of many of the experiences of childhood. Those of us who are fiercely independent as adults can only accept the experience of confused dependency associated with cancer treatment by retreating into childhood. The responsible adult with whom we identify ourselves may find the status of patient intolerable, but the child in each of us can accept it. Regression thereby enables those of us with strong needs for autonomy to delegate power to others, to place ourselves in their hands and to accept care from them. It would be exceedingly difficult to do so, even temporarily, without the safety of rediscovered childhood. Those of us with reliant temperaments turn easily toward others during periods of stress and simply experience the warm safety of the protected child. We retreat into a familiar mood of behavior and receive its benefits.

A great deal of anxiety associated with cancer is triggered by our fantasies of the future. Avoiding the future can therefore diminish these disruptive thoughts. A child's time perspective is based upon the perception of hours and days rather than months and years. By regressing into childhood, it is often possible for patients to reexperience this childlike "present tense." They can thereby find a refuge in being taken care of day by day and more easily avoid catastrophic fantasies of the future.

There are other fears that are soothed by a temporary childlike state. The cancer crisis evokes profound questions and nagging doubts. A time in which no adult responsibilities are demanded and one is simply taken care of affords the opportunity to reflect and clarify long-neglected issues. Patients have described such a time of imposed dependency as a plateau from which they were able to survey their lives. "I never had time to stop and look at myself. I raced about never giving a thought where I was racing to in such a hurry. When I got sick, it somehow seemed all right to tuck myself up under the covers and think about these things."[6] This man could not allow himself to spend time in reflective activity until his illness provided the justification. He became childlike, gave in to the process of slow recuperation and even allowed himself, for the first time in his adult life, to be pampered by others. He could allow this dependent state only through a childlike regression and only because he had just undergone cancer treatment. But he did manage to accept the care and to use the time productively to reassess the direction of his life. It is often even harder for devoted wives and nurturing mothers to permit themselves this dependent refuge in which they can reflect on the shape of their lives.

Each of us may also make use of regression during the formidable task of facing our own death. The two temperamental tendencies demonstrated by Zelda and Miriam become distinctly divergent when any of us are engaged in this task. Those with Zelda's reliant traits will continue to cling to childhood modes of behavior. They will elevate their physician to a godlike status and become more and more dependent on him. Such patients will also regard family members as peripheral to their everyday needs and may become more withdrawn from the family. The common need to make the physician all important should be respected. It is not a repudiation of the family that underlies the withdrawal but a powerful need for an authoritative parental figure. Those with Miriam's autonomous traits will respond in a very different manner. They will strive for more independence and personal authority, they will resent being "managed" and they will try to retain their active roles in family life and treatment as long as possible.

There are rare but reported instances when thought and behavior become delusional and the regressive state takes on extreme (psychotic) proportions. Doctors and nurses are accused of attempted murder, family members are believed to be hatching evil plots and vivid hallucinations accompany these imagined episodes. On such occasions, the circumstances should be carefully investigated. The images might well be exaggerated versions of real grievances. It is also helpful to curtail visits temporarily and to explain all medical procedures carefully. Family members should avoid bedside whispering. Medication might be required. But there is no cause for panic. Within a short period of time, the delusions will subside and the regression will become less ominous.

It is, however, important to remember that normal regression can be quite extreme. Some of us might gratefully let ourselves be fed and bathed. Others might have an almost insatiable hunger to be held and rocked or to sleep with a soft toy. These temporary regressions into infancy should not be discouraged. They are valid attempts to cope with stress and are often the first steps in the difficult process of adaptation. Regression provides a safe place which, when no longer needed, will be discarded. As health professionals or family members, we can do several things to make the period of regression productive. We can endeavor to respect the childlike needs of the patient and strive to preserve as much constancy as possible (in furniture, visits, the giving of medicine, the times of disturbances).

In this way we can help to create a predictable and therefore reassuring environment. An understanding of regression implies a willingness to make few demands on the patient and to remain available for his needs. It is easier to accomplish this when we remember that the state of regression is a strategy of adaptation that carries its own eventual resolution.

Guilt and the Safety of Crime and Punishment

Guilt is frequently used in an attempt to create inner quietness and a safe emotional refuge. It may at first seem paradoxical that a feeling as painful as guilt could possibly be used as a means of establishing emotional security. The strategy is complicated and usually remains beyond our awareness. But it is used by most of us and we can understand, at least in principle, the way it works.

A sense of guilt is one of the dominant aspects of the cancer crisis. Most patients have a compulsion to explain the cancer in terms of what they did or failed to do.[7] Most parents assume the blame for their child's cancer in the same manner.[8] This predominance of guilt does not, however, attend all serious illness. Heart patients, for example, do not respond to their diagnosis with self-accusation.[9] But self-condemnation is characteristic of cancer patients and their families. Cancer is irrational. It strikes at random, by chance: an innocent child, a good man, a young mother, you, me. This assault remains incomprehensible and terrifying without a framework of reward and punishment. Almost all cancer patients and their families try to make sense out of the cancer experience by seeking the origins of the disease. But why this assumption of personal responsibility? The self-referring idea is as old as time itself. "With the approach of the first winter, Adam began to see the days getting shorter. 'Woe is me,' he said, 'because I must have sinned and as a punishment the world is being darkened and returned to a state of chaos and confusion.' "[10] Adam's sense of transgression is based upon his belief that all undesirable events must necessarily derive from sinful behavior. The undesirable is defined as punishment; punishment is evidence of personal transgression; personal transgression must be identified and repented to prevent a state of chaos and confusion. Adam's archaic moral formula is busily at work in almost all of us.

Identifiable Transgressions. Many of the imagined transgressions are sexual. A young woman we will call Martha had established a secret sexual relationship with the husband of her best friend. Cancer was diagnosed and she was scheduled for surgery. On the day of admission, she was driven to the hospital by her lover and his wife. The patient was convinced that the cancer was retribution for her sexual sins and that she had been justifiably brought to the "place of punishment" by her rival.[11] Lillian, a devoutly religious woman, had cancer of the tongue. She had had an affair before her marriage with a "wild and handsome man." She was so "crazy" about him that she committed "unholy" sexual acts, including oral intercourse. She believed that God not only punished her for her sinfulness, but that in true Biblical style he punished the offending organ, her mouth, as well.[12] One woman who had a mastectomy simply blamed herself for having beautiful breasts, which she believed created jealousy in others and thereby aroused the "evil eye."[13] Other imagined transgressions involve hostility. Bessie knew exactly why she had cancer. She grew up in a poor family with four brothers whom she detested. One of them was killed in an accident. She blamed herself, "prayed to the Lord for punishment" and believed He finally answered her prayers.[14] Another woman says: "My cancer came from cursing my mother before she died."[15] Moral transgression can be defined in many ways. Martin, an Indian from southwestern California, believed that his cancer resulted from transgressing the mores of his group. He explicitly listed those sins: taking more than his share of food and keeping more money than was necessary to maintain himself and not sharing it.[16]

Many patients blame themselves, not for moral transgressions, but for conspicuous neglect. A woman says: "I failed to eat adequate amounts of food." Another says: "I was worn out caring for my mother."[17] Some patients project the cause of their cancer onto others; they locate a villain instead of blaming themselves. In doing so, they are also attempting to establish order by defining a cause of their cancer. A woman claimed that her breast tumor came from borrowing clothes (against her mother's advice) from a sister-in-law who died of cancer.[18] Another woman accused her husband of fondling her breast too much. And another said that her husband "made too many sexual demands."[19] A barber believed that his cancer was caused by the hair of a foreign man which had penetrated his finger.[20]

Very possibly the best illustration of the use of guilt as explanation for cancer is one instance in which no plausible transgression could be established. Harry could not find an acceptable sin to explain his cancer. "I never drank or whored around, I have always lived a good clean life. I don't understand why I got cancer."[21] Locating the transgression or person responsible for the affliction of cancer helps to deny the intolerable thought that no one is responsible. Were the tragic event perceived as impersonal and meaningless, it could not be undone by power of will or concept of crime sufficiently punished. To assign a guilt meaning to cancer is to regain some desperately needed measure of control and to create a safe reprieve from chaos and confusion.

The safety provided by a moral system of crime and punishment is as helpful to family members as it is for cancer patients. Investigators, in one major study of families with leukemic children, state: "Mothers consistently expressed guilt and personal responsibility about their part in the causation of the disease."[22] All family members seem to share this belief. "Laurie had an ear infection and a bad rash. The doctor waited two months before admitting he didn't know what it was. Then an allergist treated her roughly for weeks with his ridiculous tests. What a mistake I made in not stopping him. I feel so bad about it and so guilty." Her husband adds: "I thought [my wife] was just being hysterical so I told her to stop being silly and I supported the doctors. It's my fault that we didn't find out in time."[23] "I've always been nervous. Were all mothers nervous? Can that be the reason?"; "I knock myself out worrying about the times I've fussed her and wouldn't let her do things"[24]; "I had a radioactive dye test during my pregnancy and that gave him cancer.

I caused it and I was too damned stupid to catch it."[25]

The experience of guilt is a part of the desperate search for an explanation. It is poignantly expressed by this mother: "I've thought of everything I have done and everything that happened since his conception. I have to blame somebody and I don't feel I can blame my husband so I have to blame myself."[26] And by this wife: "Stan wanted to have relationships with other women and I refused. I wouldn't let him and then he got cancer. I know that's why he got cancer. He was dissatisfied with our marriage and frustrated with me and that's the way it came out."[27]

In these ways a cause is identified and chaos is transformed into deserved punishment. Even psychological understanding can be exploited. "I gave birth to twins when Willie was three years old and I was in the hospital for five days. He must have been extremely angry to have lost his mother for so long but he never said a word. He held it all inside and the stress developed into cancer. I know it did. It's my fault . . . if only I could have helped him vent his anger, he would never have gotten leukemia."[28] This mother's awareness of separation anxiety, sibling rivalry and the problems of suppressed anger have been used to convict herself of murdering her child. She did not cause her child's cancer but it will do no good to lecture her (or other cancer patients and family members) about the complex origins of cancer. We would do better to ask what benefit she derives from believing that she was responsible for her child's cancer. A part of the answer is expressed by another mother in the identical situation: "It's terrible not to know what caused it because I don't know how to protect the other children."[29] *To know* the cause is to have some power, control and effectiveness over what might happen. To have caused the cancer oneself or to have isolated its origin establishes an understandable order, and where there are order and understanding, there is also hope of resolution.

Guilt as a Source of Power. The benefits of guilt and assumed responsibility are clear indeed. One desperate father insisted that his son's cancer came from their farm animals and that he was thereby indirectly responsible for its presence. He created a diet that was completely devoid of meat, milk products and anything traceable to farm animals. He established a theory that could transform "bad blood" into "good blood."[30] This man was attempting to regain some sense of control, and the attempt required him to believe that he knew the cause and was partially responsible for his son's illness. It also required the illusion that his activities would cure cancer.

For most cancer patients, however, an identifiable transgression serves as the crime and cancer cured by effective but painful treatment is interpreted as sufficient punishment. There is a chance that the "slate has been wiped clean" if the transgression can be completely absolved through the suffering and stress of cancer. Although the imagined transgression cannot be undone, the painful repentance has the power to erase sin by permitting the sinner to undergo a moral rebirth. Marie, a devout Catholic, was only thirty-two years old when she discovered that she had a brain tumor. Her doctor believed that a pregnancy would change her hormonal balance and generate new tumor growth. He strongly recommended "foolproof birth control." Marie's husband wanted to have a vasectomy but she insisted on having a tubal ligation herself. Marie would not let him "make such a great sacrifice." Her husband said through angry tears: "It would be so much easier for me if I could do something to help. But she's got to be a martyr. She's got to do everything and keep me from doing anything to help."[31] Marie experienced the cancer as a punishment and she was determined to suffer her full measure. She could not stand to hear her husband say he loved her. She only felt receptive to further sacrifice because her secret, life-preserving hope was to suffer enough to achieve redemption. It is a painful but understandable process.

Family members, following the death of a loved one, often experience a bewildering pain known as "survivor's guilt." It derives from an irrepressible sense of triumph; from the forbidden inner exclamation "I am still alive!" There is almost always an experience of guilt at the death of a person who has been important in one's life.[32] There is so much that was said or not said, done or not done. Some of the guilt can rest upon realistic regret, and some of it has no rational justification. A great deal of post mortem hair tearing and chest beating is also an unconscious attempt to suffer and not be punished for having survived.[33]

Despite the pain engendered, our system of crime and punishment serves us well by providing a refuge from the terrifying unknown. It is used to offset the intolerable uncertainties of the cancer crisis. The system of punishment for identified transgression also offers some hope of redemption. It is a traditional and time-honored method of producing order from chaos. The Biblical story of Job is a perfect example of such an effort to account for affliction by means of assumed transgression. How else could Job explain his fall from grace? How else could his friends make sense of this "perfect" man's sudden plunge from the heights of fortune? Affliction must derive from sinful behavior. He need only discover his transgression, repent, suffer enough and reform to once again gain favor with God. In this respect, Job's friends are exactly like most of us. They use the assumption of transgression to construct an orderly system of crime and punishment, and they do so to protect themselves from the terror of universal chaos.

And yet, with time and a lessening of anxiety, most of us begin to relinquish our desperate use of guilt. We begin to acknowledge our human limitations and we begin to view cancer as a disease independent of the orderly boundaries of crime and punishment. But it is hard to desert the place of safety afforded by a moral order. Most of us can give up the benefits of denial when they are no longer needed and we simply grow out of the childlike state of regression. But it is not always easy to extricate ourselves from the powerful and intricate self-condemnations which we have adopted. In fact, these purposeful, punitive judgments are not easy to explain away even when they are no longer of any benefit. It is at this stage that an alternative interpretation of the cancer experience may serve as a bridge from self-condemnation to self-acceptance.

Blake's Vision of Job. William Blake, in his wonderful illustrations for the Book of Job, violently rejects both the argument that Job's afflictions must be a punishment for transgression against God's law and the explanation that God and Satan agreed to test Job's faith.

He believes that the story bears eloquent witness to the "vulgar error" of assuming that misfortunes are punishment for sinful transgression.[34]

According to Blake, Job is consoled at first by the belief that he has sinned, that he must endure his suffering with resignation and that sufficient sorrow will bring redemption. But he begins to rage against his suffering after an extended period of remorse and repentance. His proverbial patience comes to an end and an unfamiliar wrath bursts forth. The emotional rebellion serves as a turning point and Job begins to question the justice of his tragic circumstance. At first his rage lashes out in all directions, but then he begins to consider the values and assumptions of his life. His rage and reflection bring forth a chorus of accusations from his friends, who insist that his misfortune issues from transgression; that his blasphemous anger and questioning can only lead to greater punishment. Job rebels, rejects his friends and appeals for some other explanation. He is visited with a terrifying vision—with the very perception his assumption of guilt was designed to avoid.

Job's dark vision, as depicted by Blake, is truly terrifying: damnation, hell itself and a troop of devils reach up through sinister fire to pull him down. But the condemning God is Satan masquerading as the vengeful God of justice. Job suddenly sees that everyone could be condemned to this nightmare world because everyone is imperfect. He understands that this universal condemnation could not belong to a just God but only to Satan himself. He begins to understand that his true God offers forgiveness. Although his friends berate him for his failure to feel guilt and to repent, Job clings to his new understanding, and in the last illustration he experiences the extreme joy of understanding and acceptance.

The story of Job depicts a profound *psychological journey*. Blake himself asks us not to take his illustrations literally. The entire drama is enacted within Job's mind: his children are his deeds, his friends are guilt-ridden aspects of himself, the rebellion against his friends is his own conflict between self-condemnation and self-acceptance, his true God is the manifestation of his own ideal. The story of Job represents the struggle experienced by most of us who venture beyond the safety of the system of crime and punishment. The journey toward tolerance of inexplicable disorder can be extremely difficult. Blake's beautiful interpretation provides us with one path. His essential conviction is that our greatest sin is committed in the act of believing our inner voice of self-condemnation. Blake insists that "Job's error" was allowing the "accuser" into his life, that Job erred when he unquestioningly accepted his afflictions as just punishment, that he erred precisely at the moment he became complicit with this Satanic voice of self-condemnation. Blake was a religious man who thought in Biblical metaphor. But his psychological understanding was surprisingly contemporary. His work envisions Christ as the highest ideal precisely because Christ rejects the concept of pernicious guilt and replaces it with forgiveness.

Cancer is almost always experienced as a punishment; a punishment is almost always associated with a crime; a crime sufficiently punished is thought to be redeemable. Such understandable systems of order and control provide a safe refuge from chaos and thereby foster the process of adaptation. But there is a path of forgiveness and self-acceptance for those who elect to step beyond the system of crime and punishment. This step requires courage and great tolerance for conflict. But the struggle does lead toward the reaffirmation of oneself.

The Illusion of Omnipotence and the Limits of Responsibility

Denial and regression provide refuge by means of temporary retreat from a terrible reality. They are psychological states in which no responsibility need be assumed. The guilt system offers safety through personal responsibility, self-blame and control. However, feeling responsible for having contributed to the presence of cancer is only one of the several ways in which "being responsible" can be used to regain a sense of control. Another way to acquire emotional safety through responsibility is to assume total responsibility for everyone and everything during the cancer crisis. But the assumption of so much responsibility can only carry the promise of safety if we also secretly believe that we have limitless powers to restore order. The safety of responsibility and the illusion of omnipotence are easy to understand. Active behavior, the experience of "doing something" can be extremely reassuring. This is especially so for family members.

There is usually one member of the family who provides most of the patient's home care and emotional support. Such a person (whether spouse, child, parent, sister, brother or friend) assumes enormous responsibility and is most often plagued with self-doubts. He asks himself to attend to a patient's shifting needs, monitor contact with the world outside the home and offer protection from anything painful or disruptive. Living with doubt, grieving alone, neglecting personal needs and rejecting help are all too common. Although the assumption of total responsibility can provide a sense of control and effectiveness, some guidelines concerning the limits of responsibility are essential. The assumption of total responsibility for everything can become self-defeating for the family member and ultimately problematic for the patient.

I once worked with a couple who were caught in rigid roles: Jim was the "fragile patient," Martha the dutiful, self-sacrificing "wife-nurse." Martha was becoming increasingly frustrated and Jim felt her growing impatience. I asked him if he wanted to know what she was really experiencing.[35]

JIM: Yes, of course.
MARTHA: O.K., I'm having some trouble with this and it's been getting worse. I want to just take care of you but I'm feeling trapped in the house; I'm starting to climb the walls. I go back and forth inside. You sure you want to hear this?
JIM: Yes, go on.
MARTHA: I'm starting to resent taking care of you because I can't get out. [*What stops you?*] Jim does. He won't say don't go, but he needs me there. [*Ask him about that.*] Well, you do, don't you?
JIM: Of course I need you there, but for God's sake, not all the time. You think you have to hover over me. Go ahead, go out, see Ann, have some fun, I'll let you know if I need you.
MARTHA: Now you're hurt and angry.

JIM: Yes, I am. You're treating me like a baby. You're tiptoeing around like you don't know who I am any more. I don't like it. I'm not about to fall apart. [To Martha—*Do you believe him?*]

MARTHA: I want to. [*What are you afraid of?*] That I'll be out and he'll really need something, you know, be in trouble and I'll never forgive myself. [*And, Jim, what are you afraid of?*]

JIM: That she will do everything she thinks she's supposed to and get more and more resentful . . . until she can't stand it any more and then she'll leave for good.

Martha's conflict had more to do with her ambivalent needs than with her husband's illness. She was torn between her understandable need to take care of herself, to be away for a time, to continue living her own life, and her understandable need to love and care for her sick husband. But she also needed to feel in control of her life. Being able to talk about her conflict enabled both of them to discover how they each had participated in establishing the trap. Martha began to understand that she had assumed total responsibility for Jim's recovery and that it was hard to let go. She finally worked out a balance that felt comfortable for her. Jim was immensely relieved to discover that her impatience did not signify the rejection he feared. Discussing "shameful" feelings may seem unthinkable, but more often than not the discussion will produce relief rather than shock and dismay.

Family members can share their experiences with one another and the exchange can be an enormous benefit. At times, as with Martha, it is possible to discuss potential areas of resentment directly. When this occurs without blaming, the patient feels more involved in the process of home care and the family member is spared the burden of assuming full responsibility for everything.

When discussions of this kind are not possible with the patient, it is essential for family members to find a person who can listen empathetically to the emotional difficulties inherent in providing home care. The need to share some of the burden with another is absolutely valid. For instance, a patient might angrily attack or passively accuse the family member who assumes primary responsibility more than anyone else. The anger or despair is directed at the closest and safest available person. It is therefore extremely important for family members to anticipate such outbursts, to hear them as part of the process of adaptation (not as accurate comments about themselves) and to have someone with whom it is possible to share the strain of such circumstances.

It is also of vital importance to be able to ask for help. There are a variety of specific needs that can be met by physicians, homemakers, visiting nurses and other health professionals. Social workers can help locate and arrange for these services. So can the local units of the American Cancer Society. Assistance can be sought for simple physical needs and for complex emotional conflicts. The accelerating demands of the cancer crisis can produce a bewilderment that is best approached by seeking the help of less emotionally involved people. All related experiences and problems can be acknowledged to oneself and to others. There are people available in each of our lives who can help sort them out. The greatest obstacle lies within the person experiencing the difficulty, in the safety of the illusion of omnipotence, in the stubborn refusal to scale down expectations of oneself. I have rarely met anyone who had assumed responsibility for a cancer patient who would do more than pay lip service to his emotional limitations, who would give up his desire to solve whatever problems arose and who would accept the human boundaries of his powers of restoration. A great deal of suffering can emerge from these self-directed demands for omnipotence. I ask you to consider this point more deeply and by means of the following illustration.

Some years ago I was a seminar leader for an interdisciplinary group of health professional students. Each week we would be presented with a difficult clinical problem and then discuss its many ramifications. I have never forgotten one presentation or the response it evoked in all of us. A renowned surgeon came before us and said: "Two years ago I received a letter from a mother in Brazil. Her son was dying of kidney disease and his sister had offered one of her kidneys if I would perform the transplant. After reviewing the records I agreed. Unfortunately, the sister's kidney was rejected. I was able to find some available time for the boy on a research kidney dialysis machine. Another transplant attempt failed and I then discovered that he had a rare white cell type that required a specific donor. The blood tests for the screening are enormously expensive." At this point in his presentation the surgeon introduced us to the young man. The patient briefly described how much he wanted to live and how hard the uncertain wait was for him.

The surgeon continued: "A woman offered us one of her kidneys. She did not know the patient but was eager to be a donor as her health was excellent and the likelihood of suffering kidney disease in her remaining kidney after surgery was remote. Unfortunately, she had the wrong white cell type and we could not accept her offer." He then introduced the woman to us. She was a warm, intelligent and articulate person. She said that she was very disappointed and would be willing to donate her kidney to another patient if the need arose.

The surgeon continued: "So here is my problem, here is the patient, here is the need. Their visitors' visas have expired and the immigration people are demanding that the family return to Brazil even though this means that the boy will die. They have run out of money, the temporary dialysis arrangement which keeps him alive is almost completed and I'm not sure I can locate another. Is anyone here willing to donate one of your kidneys to help him?" No one volunteered.

The members of my seminar all experienced the same conflict. We were unwilling to give a stranger, no matter how needy or sympathetic, one of our kidneys. And yet, on another level, we all felt that we should be willing to do so. We resented being put in such an uncomfortable position and forced to experience our rejection of his appeal. The discussion that followed demonstrated that we were *incapable* of envisioning circumstances in which we could refuse an appeal for help (especially help we could provide) without feeling guilty and selfish. There were limits to our willingness to sacrifice but the accompanying self-recrimination was evidence that there were no limits to our sense of responsibility. A voice within each of us seemed to say: "Never mind all the reasons for declining; you should be willing to give whatever benefits a person in distress." The discussion was a crucial one for young health professionals embark-

ing on a career of service; they came to realize that, if they chose to
lead lives based upon other principles in addition to those of self-
sacrifice, they would at times have to say No to the appeals of others
in need. In other words, a part of them would always demand that
they assume responsibility for all suffering and attempt to resolve it.
But a larger part, a part they also respected and hoped to keep in
perspective, would ask for a balance that also included their personal
needs and would demand the right to say No. They came to understand that this choice meant they were asking themselves to experience the predictable guilt that was bound to follow such a choice.

I believe all of us face these choices and that we all have the ability
to establish a reasonable balance for ourselves. The cancer crisis puts
this ability to the test. Assuming total responsibility for another and
pretending to the illusion of omnipotence can be enormously useful
and it can offer an emotional refuge. It can also, when rigidly maintained, become another unnecessary burden. The word responsibility is derived from the Latin words *re* (thing or circumstance) and
pono (to put in place). Being responsible is indeed knowing where
to place things, knowing the appropriate boundaries of one's capacities and then fulfilling those human expectations. The need to create
a balance between service and personal need cannot be stressed too
strongly, for it is the achievement of such a balance that permits most
people to express their full devotion.

6

The Maintenance of Personal Authority

I shall be telling this with a sigh
Somewhere ages and ages hence:
Two roads diverged in a wood, and I—
I took the one less traveled by,
And that has made all the difference.
                                    —ROBERT FROST

Worthiness and Competence

I have illustrated some divergent approaches to the task of establishing emotional stability during the cancer crisis. But all of us, regardless of other temperamental requirements, share the need for self-esteem. To confront a crisis without self-esteem is to be hopelessly adrift and to experience oneself as naked and defenseless. None of us can be indifferent to the way in which we judge ourselves. The presence or absence of self-esteem has great impact on our experience of life, our behavior and even on our perceptions of the world. A man who esteems himself feels warmth and gratitude when another expresses affection for him. A man with little self-esteem doubts the authenticity of affection offered.

The diagnosis of cancer is often experienced as an assault on one's sense of personal worth. A patient's self-esteem is often wounded by the discovery that he is seriously ill, and the feeling of vulnerability that accompanies this loss of self-esteem is particularly painful and problematic during the cancer crisis. Everyone attempts to regain a positive sense of himself. Once again, those with reliant temperaments differ conspicuously from those with autonomous temperaments in how they hope to reestablish their besieged sense of self-worth—in how they go about the task of retaining a favorable estimate of themselves.

Self-esteem presupposes a conviction that one is both *worthy* to live and *competent* to survive successfully.[1] Each of us silently judges whether or not we are worthy of life. The origins and the standards for this value judgment can range from the secular to the religious, from the rational to the irrational, from the life-affirming to the life-denying. But, regardless of origin, our feeling of personal self-worth depends on whether or not we live up to these standards. In addition to worthiness, each of us judges whether or not we have the authority and the personal effectiveness to deal with the world. This sense of personal competence exists when we approve the manner in which we make decisions and possess an inner assurance that it is possible to do what is necessary to survive. Although both subjective assessments (worthiness and competence) are important parts of self-esteem, those with dominant tendencies toward reliance are more concerned with feeling worthy, while those with dominant tendencies toward autonomy are more preoccupied with their sense of competence.

The following chapter will deal with the latter source of self-esteem—the preservation of personal competence and the maintenance of personal authority. It is intended primarily for those with autonomous temperaments. In it we shall see that there are two primary ways in which personal authority can be vigorously retained: one can participate in the decisions of cancer treatment and one can affect the actual process of physical healing.

The Core of Personal Competence

An infant acquires a sense of personal effectiveness by exerting a growing influence over his environment. His sense of competence matures slowly through the success of this ongoing struggle. But the judgment remains within him. "In his attempts to walk, the child is apt to have an appreciative audience . . . but he does not have to have approval in order to know that he has succeeded. Mind and muscles have been pitted against an unknown but unmistakable force that tries to pull him to the floor, and they have proved competent to triumph over this force."[2] The infant does not have to be told he has succeeded. He does not have to compare his success to that of others. The goal is self-generated and the self-defined accomplishment is a personal gratification.

The sense (or absence) of personal competence begins as a purely inner judgment. Although the approval or disapproval of others can often replace this inner sense, the capacity to determine one's competence remains intact and can be reestablished. It is always possible to take counsel within oneself and formulate criteria of one's own choosing. It is possible to refer to such personal standards and decline those suggested by others.

Charles[3] had major cancer surgery and was up and about within three days despite his family's desperate pleas that he remain in bed. He designed special exercises and actually built a swimming pool during his "recuperation." Charles had a lifelong interest in body fitness and preserved his sense of competence by once again *proving* his physical prowess. Jenny[4] set a totally different task for herself; she elected to let go. She had been an active woman who had always been able to "berate" anyone who stood in her way in order to achieve her ends. She wanted now to do what she had never done in her life; she wanted to *surrender* to the experience of cancer treatment; she wanted to learn to trust herself enough to let go of her need to "control everything." These two cancer patients are both attempting to sustain their sense of personal competence and they are approaching their tasks in almost diametrically opposing ways. Charles's behavior asserts that he is unconquerable. Jenny's behavior asserts that she is capable of surrender. Each is attempting to reach a goal of his own choosing and each will judge his success accordingly. Given their different perspectives, they might strongly disapprove of each other's behavior. Charles might criticize her for giving up and being a coward. Jenny could easily be critical of him for foolishly refusing to accept his temporary physical limitations. But their disapproval would be irrelevant. The feeling of personal competence can only be realized through appropriately selected personal goals.

And yet, what if Charles had not been physically able to get out of bed? What if Jenny had not been emotionally capable of surrendering control? Would their self-esteem have plummeted? It would do so only if they mistook their lack of success with a specific task for an overall assessment of their capacity to be effective. Charles and Jenny, one hopes, experience pride and continued self-esteem as a result of their demonstrated capacity to succeed. Correspondingly, they will feel no pride if they fail to achieve their goals. But their overall capacity to be effective human beings should not be impaired. Self-esteem ought never to depend upon a specific success or failure. And this is especially true during the cancer crisis, when there are so many factors that lie beyond the patient's volitional control. Goals must be constantly reevaluated; what we attempt to do must be carefully reconsidered in the light of new developments. Our sense of self-esteem cannot be allowed to rise and fall with the success or failure of every attempted task. Self-esteem is established over a long period of time. It is the product of many choices, behaviors and accomplishments. It is the "overall reputation a man acquires with himself."[5] Once achieved, self-esteem cannot be maintained automatically but it should never depend upon the experience of infallibility; we must not allow it to collapse as a consequence of a single mistake or honest failure.

Mature self-esteem resides in the capacity to clarify opportunities and comprehend what we need, rather than with the adolescent notion of limitless accomplishment. Everyone feels inferior in a great many ways, but self-esteem is dependent upon only a small area of competence. William James described his self-esteem in this circumscribed manner: "I, who for the time have staked my all on being a Psychologist, am mortified if others know much more of Psychology than I. But I am content to wallow in the grossest ignorance of Greek. My deficiencies there give me no sense of personal humiliation at all . . . our self feeling in this world depends entirely upon what we *back* ourselves to be and do."[6]

All of us choose goals and tasks. Our sense of personal authority and competence is reflected in these choices and we are free to alter any decision that becomes unrealistic. It is certainly possible to derive self-esteem from our ability to shift toward more appropriate tasks when those we have undertaken seem to elude us.

One woman who had always secured great pleasure from the shape of her beautiful breasts insists that the mastectomy has destroyed all hope of future happiness. She claims that the surgery has stripped away all possibilities of experiencing esteem for herself. Another woman, equally proud of her breasts, mourns the loss of her body integrity and begins to develop other aspects of herself. She believes that she has experienced a great deal during the cancer crisis and has gained in wisdom, compassion and strength. By accepting the development of these qualities as an admirable goal, she grows in stature, becomes more of a woman in her own eyes and experiences an expansion of personal competence and self-worth.

A crisis often forces us to experience the core of our personal competence. The woman who grew in wisdom and strength described a stressful experience that led to this discovery: "The time in the hospital when I lost my breast was horrible, just horrible. [*What do you think sustained you?*] I know what it was—a specific event. It happened a long time ago and in a funny way it has something to do with what we were just talking about. I was in my twenties and very unhappy. I was walking on a country road. I felt like I couldn't go on. It was awful. I wasn't going to kill myself but I felt as though the whole thing I was facing was absolutely impossible. There was no way I could get out, no way I could breathe, no way I could understand, there was no way I could do anything. So I walked and I walked and came to a meadow with some trees in it. I don't even know why I decided to go there and rest among the trees but I did. And as I sat there I had this fantastic feeling. It's impossible to put in words but the closest would be—'I have myself; I have something in me.' That feeling has never left me completely. That's what I have that sustained me and I don't even know what it is."[7]

I would interpret this event as the discovery of a deep-seated sense of self-esteem. It is the product of an underlying feeling that one is personally capable of facing difficulties, personally capable of understanding them, personally competent to attend to them and therefore worthy of the right to determine one's fate through choice.*

Personal Competence and Choice

There is a tendency in each of us to view those events that determine the direction of our lives as external and unalterable. There are those for whom this tendency has grown into an exclusive perception. They insist that their choices are unnecessary, that, in fact, there really is no choice, that necessity dictates. Those of us who adopt this perspective deny the fact that we have chosen to do what we have done. All women who have biopsies of their breast must decide whether or not to give the surgeon permission to perform a mastectomy if the biopsy is positive. They must make a choice in advance of knowing. There are as many women who prefer to have it all done at once as there are women who prefer to have only the biopsy. The latter (48 percent) want to have surgery when they "know what to expect, have time to think and a chance to talk."[8]

Each woman possesses the same potential alternatives and each is making a choice. Each is deciding how she wishes to proceed. Those who choose to prepare themselves for radical surgery, who choose to engage themselves in such issues as the type of surgery and the background and qualifications of the surgeon, will experience the difficult conflicts and weighty responsibilities of their active participation. Those who choose to have the doctor decide for them will usually insist that if surgery is necessary it's necessary, and if it's necessary they really have no choice. But, in fact, they have all chosen. The decisive factor is the ability to tolerate conflict and thereby gain an awareness of choice. "The greater our tolerance the more freedom we retain, the less our tolerance the more we jettison;

---

*The examples presented in Part One were meant to illustrate the wide range of stressful experiences associated with cancer. However, the examples presented in the rest of the book are meant to illustrate possible resolutions and life-affirming approaches to this stress.

for high among the uses of necessity is relief from tension. What we can't alter we don't have to worry about; so the enlargement of necessity is a measure of economy in psychic housekeeping. The more issues we have closed the fewer we have to fret about."[9]

The choices of the cancer crisis are often limited. We cannot choose to be free of cancer. And yet there are some respects in which cancer patients are much less limited than others. Heart disease usually leads to permanent physical impairment. Cancer patients, following their convalescence, often encounter no permanent physical restrictions to work or play. However, it is not the number of alternatives we have but the process of active choice that sustains our sense of personal competence. The number of potential alternatives does not determine whether or not one experiences a choice. Escape from the freedom of choice into the determined world of necessity is always a great temptation. It takes courage to abandon voluntarily the safe role of victim. It takes courage to experience the inevitable doubts and conflicts that are a part of assuming personal responsibility for that which is possible. It takes courage to perceive one's choices.

Conflict and anxiety are not the failure of confidence; they are the price of assuming one's right to choose. A patient says: "The doctor gave me a choice of four possible treatments. It was horrible. If it didn't work out then it was my fault. I had demanded to know but I didn't want to feel responsible."[10] This patient had not realized that assuming personal responsibility included the experience of anxiety, doubt and conflict. Nor had the physician who said: "Is this being unfair . . . to ask [a patient] to help make a life or death decision that we physicians have to make on inadequate evidence anyway?"[11] But the question of fairness is irrelevant. Some patients and some family members prefer to participate, knowing they will experience greater conflict, doubt and anxiety because of their participation. Other patients and family members choose to have the physician retain full authority for these decisions and to remain within the safer range of what is necessary. It is my opinion that the right to participate in the important decisions of one's life is of special significance when there is "inadequate evidence"! It is precisely under these circumstances that our decisions must reflect a wide range of issues, values and preferences. The right to choose becomes more precious when the choices are difficult and the context unclear.

Although the range of free choice is often smaller with cancer than with other diseases, our ability to influence the course of events, and the experience of these events, is immense. Consider some other aspects of life which are even less susceptible to personal influence than life-threatening disease. We age and eventually die; we watch our children mature to independence and grow beyond our control; we live with inflation and crime. None of us can personally arrest any of these forces, but we have an important sphere of influence within them and a great many potential choices. If we approach the process of aging with acceptance rather than terrified malice, aging can become a meaningful part of our lives. And, if we attend to diet, grooming and dress, the process can be both dignified and attractive. If we offer nurturance and support to our children, and when they come of age accept the inappropriateness of attempting to control their behavior, we will have influenced their lives through the example of our own maturity. Inflation and crime cannot be eliminated by any behavior issuing from a single individual. But we are all capable of proceeding with care and discretion and of minimizing the personal impact of these potential disasters.

The same range of choice and influence is available to all cancer patients and their families. One patient lies in a hospital bed feeling outraged about but helpless to change the inconsiderate manner in which he is being treated. He laments that there is nothing he can do to change his dehumanized state. Another man, who occupies a bed in the next room, crosses the hospital corridor, enters a conference room and angrily scolds the assembled doctors for discussing his case where he can hear every word they say.[12] In doing so, he has chosen to maintain his personal authority and to remain in charge of his life. One mother refused to accept her daughter's illness and felt overwhelmed by the procedures of cancer treatment. Months went by and she felt helpless and confused by everything. Another mother, who lived in the same town and found herself in the same circumstance, reestablished a sphere of choice. "If an IV ran out, I learned how to replace it. When my daughter asked about death I was prepared and could talk honestly with her. At first I was terrified but I learned a lot."[13] Each of us is capable of adopting this attitude and of maintaining a sense of personal authority.

The distinction between "I cannot accept cancer" and "I choose not to accept cancer" is crucial. To realize that one *chooses not* to accept illness (or its consequences) is to realize that one continues to have a choice. And to perceive the full range of one's possible choices is to be free to shape one's current reality. Freedom of choice cannot be taken from us; the freedom to choose is what we *are*. Even in the most difficult of circumstances there are many alternatives and there is always an area that lies within our sphere of personal influence.

Confronting Sacred Routine

The assumption of personal authority can antagonize those who depend upon undisrupted routines. Questions, personal requests, almost anything that calls for doing things differently may be met with rigid disapproval, and patients who insist upon retaining their sense of personal authority can become quite unpopular. They are confronted with a variety of subtle (and not so subtle) accusations and are made to feel ashamed for not being like "normal" and "satisfied" and "likable" patients.

Family routines can be as rigid as hospital procedures. Morton had been married for almost fifty years when his wife became a cancer patient. He was the family patriarch and a man who had always had everything done for him. He began learning how to take care of himself when it seemed obvious that she would not recover. His adaptive response embraced an effort to become more knowledgeable about "practical things" and less dependent on others. But his daughter was outraged. She anticipated taking care of him as her mother had always done and disapproved of his "silly putterings." A family struggle began when his twenty-five-year-old granddaughter came for a visit. She stayed with him and supported his attempt at domestic independence. He wanted to go to the laundromat and be shown what soaps to use. His granddaughter took him but his daughter was furious at her for not "doing grandpa's clothes." He fixed breakfast for his great-grandchildren every morning. They were delighted but his daughter was enraged: "You let him wait on the kids when grandma is sick and he's so worried." He didn't know how to care for grandma's delicate porcelain statuettes and his granddaughter showed him how to use a feather duster. His daughter was beside herself with anger.[14]

Here is a family experiencing the disruption of the cancer crisis. But in this case grandpa is choosing life. He is expanding his range of personal competence. He is preparing himself for the future and doing it in a way that meets his needs. But he is also breaking a rigid family pattern by emerging from the role of a domestically dependent child and is therefore encountering the wrath of his daughter, who wants to assume responsibility for him.

Sacred routines that surround patients are even more rigidly enforced by hospital staff. The need to emerge from the position of dependency and the need to regain a sense of personal authority is experienced by many patients and family members. "When Danny was first diagnosed, I felt the doctors were gods, you know, unapproachable. Then one said he wouldn't do a bone marrow test with me in the room. He tried to kick me out. I insisted on staying. I told him I had a trust with Danny and I wouldn't break it. I even insisted upon another doctor and got one. This doctor did the test with me there as always and, you know, my insisting was a very important moment for me. It still is."[15] Once again, a family member has chosen to maintain the right to participate in (and thereby influence) the course of cancer treatment. This mother chose to disrupt an arbitrary routine, was willing to withstand some abuse and is still experiencing the profound importance of that choice.

Some of the most painful struggles take place between patient and physician. Rose Kushner[16] insisted on participating in the decisions of cancer treatment but that preference turned into a prolonged battle. "In most instances, in this country, a woman going to sleep for a simple biopsy does not know whether she will wake up with two breasts or one. To me, not to know beforehand, what was going to happen was unthinkable . . . my lump was tiny and I was no surgical risk. I made up my mind to have a biopsy first and then wait." She began to call the surgeons recommended by her internist. " 'No patient is going to tell me how to do my surgery,' one of them growled when I asked for a two-stage operation—biopsy now, mastectomy later. 'If the diagnosis is positive on frozen section, the breast must come off immediately.' And so it went. I had been naive." Having encountered such antagonism in her attempt to locate a surgeon who would agree to perform only the biopsy, she wanted to be reassured. "With the help of a lawyer, I drafted a legalistic document to be counter-signed by the surgeon before my operation, refusing to authorize him or the hospital to do anything more than a biopsy . . . my surgeon treated the contract as a huge joke, signing it with a flourish as I watched from my stretcher. Afterward he was not so flippant. He seemed to take my refusal to let him do the mastectomy as a personal insult."

The biopsy was positive and additional treatment was required. Rose Kushner, having researched the literature on breast surgery, preferred not to have the radical Halsted procedure. She made an appointment with a top breast cancer specialist at Memorial Sloan-Kettering Cancer Center in New York, but he would only discuss the Halsted. She next went to Roswell Park Memorial Institute in Buffalo and there finally found a breast cancer specialist who would discuss various treatment procedures with her and who was willing to perform the less radical surgery if, after tests, it seemed medically sound. The tests were encouraging and an appointment for surgery was arranged. "Suddenly, surprisingly, hilariously, being able to have a mastectomy, became good news." Rose Kushner maintained her personal authority throughout this long and stressful ordeal and certainly did influence the course of her cancer treatment.

There are many instances in which a patient clearly seeks inappropriate treatment. But there are also many instances in which a patient is simply opposing a physician's arbitrary preference and rigid routine. To insist upon one's right to a voice in the decisions of treat-

ment can evoke a powerful struggle for control. An obvious alternative to this bitter struggle is an open discussion between doctor and
patient. Mutual respect fosters a healing alliance. I have emphasized
how important it is for some patients to participate actively in the
treatment process despite the many obstacles erected by health
professionals. Actively discussing the deeper issues of one's life with
family members can be just as significant.

The Opportunities of Conversation

An accepting conversation offers each of us the opportunity to
explain, to forgive, to be forgiven. It can comfort and allow the
expression of what is most feared, loved and valued; it can dissipate
the pain of loneliness and foster beauty and meaning; it can nurture
and validate the rebirth of one's spirit and one's humanity. Secrets
nearly always lead to shame and despair. Protecting someone's feelings by holding silence rarely works unless the person is deaf, dumb
and blind. Misunderstandings result and all too often actually intensify the painful emotions. The cancer crisis is notorious for its ability
to disrupt the normal channels of communication. Patients and family members withdraw in the face of uncertainty and fear; a vicious
circle of misunderstanding, discomfort, awkwardness and angry
withdrawal settles over the lives of all involved. Each of us is capable
of nurturing old, childish expectations; of saying to ourselves: "If
they truly love me, they should know how I feel and should know
what I need without my having to tell them." Children expect this
of their parents, adults all too often mistakenly expect it of each
other. Given the infinite variety of responses to identical circumstances, it is essential that we explain what we are experiencing and
what we desire to the important people in our lives. It is true that
many of us are highly intuitive, that we come to know and understand each other well, that we accurately anticipate the feelings and
actions of others. But we are not mindreaders, we possess no infalli-
ble crystal balls and we make grievous errors of interpretation.
Communicating experience is not easy. It is especially prone to

distortion during the stressful cancer crisis. Even the most sincere attempts, efforts devoid of accusation or manipulation, can fail. The message sent is not the message received. At times, descriptions of experience must be repeated over and over again; what is heard must be checked with what was said, checked and rechecked until finally it is clearly understood. Although this process is frustrating and often disheartening, the achievement of a mutual, empathetic understanding is certainly worth the effort involved. However, an individual's need for silence must take precedence over another's desire for open communication. Whenever any of us elects to remain silent about our own experience, that choice ought to be honored. In terms of personal competence, there is a great deal of difference between the active silence of choice and the passive silence of helplessness.

The Right to Die

There are few choices more controversial than those involving the right to die. There are questions of suicide and questions of life-sustaining mechanical devices and situations in which doctors or family members must decide for a comatose patient. But, given the slow progression of most cancers, there is usually time for cancer patients to deliberate, time for them to decide whether or not they want heroic procedures, time for them to choose the price they want to pay for continued life. Many people would deny patients the right to refuse treatment and the right to take their lives. Hospitals devote great effort not only to curing patients but to preventing them from killing themselves.

Many reasons are offered to justify these policies. Some are religious in nature, some contain hope for recovery, some simply assert the state's right to determine who lives and who dies. But what of the human being at the heart of such decisions? An old man makes his physician promise that she will not use heroic procedures to prolong his life. Hospital policies, however, force her to do so and many appliances are attached to his body. One day she enters his room and finds him dead. He has managed to pull out every needle and to scrawl a note: "Death is not the enemy, doctor; humanity is."[17] I do not believe that any official has the moral authority to deny this man—or any man even in the absence of illness—the right to forgo additional personal suffering. For me the issue is clear. Our life is our own possession. It is ours to preserve and it is ours to surrender. The choice for life or death cannot rest with doctors, families or the government. Freedom of choice is our greatest human endowment and that freedom must extend to life itself. Kübler-Ross expresses the concept succinctly: "If a terminally ill patient has accepted his own finiteness and has put his house in order and then wants to terminate his life, we cannot prevent it and we should not judge his decision."[18]

There are many instances in which a patient is depressed and suicidal. His awareness of choice and his range of freedom have diminished. The rejection of life is then a symptom of depression and we must all try to help such patients beyond their despair. But there are also instances in which the patient's acceptance of death has outgrown the comprehension of physician and family. In these cases, the insistence upon further desperate treatment is a coercive restriction of the patient's free choice. It is not the doctor's province to judge the value of any life but his own: the final judgment must continue to reside within each of us.

Our range of choice can expand or contract. It can be fostered or frustrated by individuals, policies or institutions. But our awareness of potential alternatives remains the most important determining factor. Those of us who wish to retain our sense of personal authority must know what to expect, think about what we might do, anticipate how we will proceed and where we will seek assistance. These needs are as common and as valid for family members as they are for cancer patients, and they span the entire treatment process. A diagnosis is made and a course of treatment is presented. There is no way to be prepared for such dreadful information. The right to ask questions at the beginning of treatment is therefore essential. Many patients need to know why certain procedures have been recommended. Even if the physician believes no alternative treatment possibilities exist, patients and their families have every right to question him, to clarify their thoughts and feelings and to seek additional consultation. Consultation is an important and accepted part of medical practice. Physicians should help make the necessary arrangements. Seeking the opinions of other experts is extremely important for many people. It allows a broader choice of possible treatment plans. And, even where treatment recommendations are identical, selecting the most trustworthy and reassuring doctor can afford a greater sense of personal authority.

In the past, the physician had absolute authority to determine what information and, to some extent, what choices a patient had. Reach to Recovery volunteers, for example, were not allowed to leave information without the physician's permission. In recent years, however, the recipients of health-care services, like all consumers, have become more assertive and have demanded a greater participation. The Reach to Recovery organization is now moving toward a policy which asserts that every mastectomy patient, with or without her doctor's permission, has the right to decide whether she wishes to talk with a Reach to Recovery volunteer.[19] The general trend toward greater choice is supported by many distinguished nurses and social workers. "More and more of us . . . are questioning whether we can continue as we did in the past, to leave all communication about the diagnosis and prognosis to the doctor . . . it appears to me that there are times when a patient cannot wait for the 'appropriate' informer, but wants to take the opportunity to share her anxieties with whom she chooses at the time she wishes to do so."[20] I applaud this trend, for it enlarges the sphere of personal influence. It is up to all of us to assert our absolute right to humanize cancer treatment whenever possible.

These rights are guaranteed. The American Civil Liberties Union has published an excellent book on the legal rights of hospitalized patients. It provides a variety of answers to questions involving issues of admission, discharge, informed consent, refusing treatment, consultation, referral and rights to confidentiality and privacy.[21] The Living Will is another simple and direct means of retaining control over one's life.[22]

Actively Influencing the Disease Cancer

Attitude and Tumor Growth. It is becoming more and more apparent that it is possible to inhibit actual tumor growth and decrease bodily incapacitation by means of voluntary personal intent. In the following pages I hope to substantiate this extremely controversial statement.

Seymour and Tony were diagnosed as having identical lung cancers with metastasis to the brain.[23] They were almost the same age, had almost identical physical conditions and received the same medical treatment. But the likeness ends with these similarities, for they had strikingly different emotional responses to their disease. Seymour did not miss a day's work (except for specific treatment procedures) during the year following his diagnosis. He began spending more time with his family and proceeded to rediscover his life. "You know," he once said, "I'd forgotten that I didn't look at the trees. I hadn't been looking at the trees and the grass and the flowers for a long time. And now I do that." He continued to get stronger and healthier each week and still continues to improve.

Tony, on the other hand, stopped working the day he received his diagnosis. He was in constant pain and had "absolutely no energy." He sat before the TV and watched the clock, so that he might remind his wife when to give him pain medication. It did no good. He suffered greatly and died within a short time. These two men had dramatically different attitudes toward their disease. Seymour turned toward life, Tony toward death.

The dangers and the opportunities of the cancer crisis offer themselves to each of us. We cannot change the diagnosis but we can *choose* the attitude with which we will deal with it. Seymour and Tony demonstrate extremely divergent attitudes. Could their attitudes and dispositions have affected the clinical course of their cancer?

Let us consider another case of a patient with advanced cancer. Although he died of his disease, his history suggests a considerable degree of emotional and attitudinal influence over the disease process of cancer.

A noted oncologist (cancer specialist)[24] reports the following case:

> Mr. Wright had a generalized far advanced lymphosarcoma. . . . He had developed resistance to all known palliative treatments. . . . Huge tumor masses the size of oranges were in the neck, axillas, groin, chest and abdomen. The spleen and liver were enormous. . . . Mr. Wright was not without hope, even though his doctors most certainly were. The reason for this was that the new drug he had expected to come along and save the day had already been reported in the newspapers. Its name was Krebiozen.
>
> Then he heard in some way that our clinic was to be one of a hundred places chosen by the American Medical Association for evaluation of this treatment. . . . Mr. Wright was not considered eligible, since one stipulation was that the patient must have a life expectancy of at least three and preferably six months [and] to give him a prognosis of more than two weeks seemed to be stretching things. When he heard we were going to begin treatment with Krebiozen, his enthusiasm knew no bounds, and as much as I tried to dissuade him, he begged so hard for this golden opportunity, that against my better judgment, and against the rules of the Krebiozen committee, I decided I would have to include him.
>
> I had left him febrile, gasping for air, completely bedridden. Now, here he was (after three days) walking around the ward, chatting happily with the nurses, and spreading his message of good cheer to any one who would listen. . . . The tumor masses had melted like snowballs on a hot stove and, in only these few days, they were half their original size. (No other patient in the study showed any improvement after treatment with Krebiozen.)
>
> The injections were given three times weekly as planned. Much to the joy of the patient, but much to our bewilderment, within ten days he was able to be discharged from his "death bed," practically all signs of his disease having vanished in this short time. . . . Within two months conflicting reports began to appear in the news, all of the testing clinics reporting no results [and] this disturbed our Mr. Wright considerably as the weeks wore on. . . . His faith waned and after two months of practically perfect health, he relapsed to his original state. . . . Deliberately lying, I told him not to believe what he read in the papers, the drug was really most promising after all. What then, he asked, was the reason for his relapse? "Just because the substance deteriorates on standing," I replied. "A new super refined double strength product is due to arrive tomorrow which can more than reproduce the great benefits derived from the original injections."

This news came as a great revelation to him, and Mr. Wright, ill as he was, became his optimistic self again, eager to start over. . . . With much fanfare and putting on quite an act (which I deemed permissible under the circumstances), I administered the first injection of the doubly potent, fresh preparation (consisting of fresh water and nothing more). The results of this experiment were quite unbelievable to us. . . . Recovery from his second near terminal state was even more dramatic than the first. Tumor masses melted, chest fluid vanished and he became ambulatory. . . . He then remained symptom free for over two months. At this time the formal AMA announcement appeared in the press—"Nation Wide Tests Show Krebiozen to Be a Worthless Drug in the Treatment of Cancer." Within a few days of this report, Mr. Wright was readmitted to the hospital . . . hope vanished and he succumbed in less than two days.

These examples suggest that attitude and emotion can have a profound influence on disease processes. There are well over two hundred scientific articles in the medical literature on the correlation between emotion and serious illness, and there is an overwhelming consensus that a significant relationship does exist. A relationship between emotion and cancer is also well documented.[25] In fact, the idea that emotion and attitude can affect the body's ability to heal and resist new tumor growth is becoming a part of modern scientific thought.

I personally have observed cancer patients who have undergone successful treatment and were living and well for years. Then an emotional stress (death of a loved one, infidelity, long unemployment) seem to have been precipitating factors in the reactivation of their disease which resulted in death. . . . There is solid evidence that the course of disease in general is affected by emotional distress. . . . It is my sincere hope that we can widen [our] quest to include the distinct possibility that within one's mind is a power capable of exerting forces which can either enhance or inhibit the progress of this disease [cancer].

These observations and hopes were expressed by Dr. Eugene P. Pendergrass in his presidential address to the American Cancer Society in 1959.

The "quest" for a deeper understanding of the emotional and attitudinal influence on cancer has yielded many encouraging developments. The new approaches are not replacements for traditional medical treatment. They augment what medicine has to offer and they can significantly modify the experience of helpless passivity reported by so many cancer patients. They can establish an experience of active and effective personal participation in cancer treatment.

Each of us has the potential to influence personally the experience of cancer and, in many cases, even to arrest tumor growth. It is not rare for motivated patients to find they can indeed reduce suffering, pain and despair. Such attitudes demand a great deal of direct personal responsibility and courage—they are for those of us with strong independent traits, for those who welcome new opportunities to assert their effectiveness. Before describing the best-known of these approaches, I want to discuss *how* attitude and emotional well-being can dramatically influence the clinical course of cancer. And, since these ideas suggest a "partnership" with health professionals, I also want to portray an encompassing concept of the doctor-patient relationship—a concept that once existed, was then forgotten, and is once again emerging in our approach to illness.

Resistance to Cancer. One of the worst feelings of the cancer crisis is the sense of having no capacity to help eliminate the cancer. But this experience and the image of cancer as an evil invader are in conflict with another reality: we *all* have cancer many times during our lifetime and our body is unaffected. Our body is usually quite capable of eliminating the malignant cells.[26] Over 80 percent of the women with carcinoma in situ (a "mild" form of cancer) in one large study required *no treatment.* They were closely followed by their physicians and their cancers were "self-controlled." The authors conclude: "All of us may have had, have or will have some form of cancer, but because of our inherent natural control of the neoplastic process [cancer] we will never know it."[27] Cancer is neither an infectious disease nor an "invader." It is a tumor formed of our own cells when they begin to multiply faster than the surrounding tissues. Our body has the capacity to speed up cell production (as in normal healing) and to slow it down. It also has the ability to eliminate malformed and useless cells. Cancer, which occurs many times in our lifetime, becomes a disease when the immune mechanisms fail to protect the body from its own tissue-producing capacity.

Many isolated factors affect our ability to resist the undesirable proliferation of cells. There are many kinds of cancer and many identifiable causes. Some, such as smoking, chronic irritation, over-exposure to sunlight, radiation and certain chemicals, are environmental. Certain viruses have been traced to the development of cancer. But it is a fact that only a few of those exposed to any of these external factors develop cancer. It is also a fact that members of certain families seem more susceptible to cancer than members of other families. The various causes of cancer are not within the scope of this book or the expertise of its author. I am concerned with helping every individual to deal more effectively with the stress of the cancer crisis. But the fact that some people who have relatively curable cancers die so quickly while others who have much less treatable cancers manage to recover their full strength and healthy vitality seems to have a great deal to do with their attitudes toward the stress of cancer. And the fact that one person with a particular cancer is immobilized by pain while another with the same tumor leads an active and meaningful life is also well within my area of concern. I believe that many of us possess the capacity to *influence* the disease process itself. It is strange and a little frightening to think of cancer this way. Dr. Pendergrass asked his membership to consider the "distinct possibility that within one's mind is a power capable of exerting forces which can either enhance or inhibit" the progress of tumor growth. That was 1959. This power has been demonstrated in a variety of settings. I ask you to consider it with me.

The most detailed and documented studies of the mind's power to influence the physical functions of the body are those involving biofeedback. The principle is quite simple. A bodily function such as heart rate, skin temperature or electrical impulse is measured, monitored and demonstrated to the person. Usually one can see a dial or hear a sound that indicates what is happening. Within a short period of time, most of us can learn to make our hearts beat faster or slower, raise or lower our blood pressure, produce more of a specific kind of brain wave or alter the electrical discharge of a single nerve cell.[28] Almost all of us are capable of achieving these changes, of modifying bodily functions of which we are hardly aware. No magic, mystery or mystical state is involved. The biofeedback equipment simply enables us to be minutely aware of what our bodies are doing and with this awareness to influence their physical functioning. The mind's power to bring about these changes has been carefully documented.

It is not yet possible to monitor the body's defense mechanisms. It is not yet possible to measure the body's normal capacity to resist tumor growth. But there is little doubt that this function (like heart rate, blood pressure, brain-wave production and cellular metabolism) can be influenced by the mind through the body's hormonal systems.[29] There is little doubt that those who continue to live despite their poor prognoses, that those who suffer less and accomplish more than could possibly be expected, and that all of those who experience successful treatment are *enhancing* their body's capacity to resist tumor growth and to heal itself.[30] Becoming a partner in one's own cancer treatment, becoming an active participant in one's own recovery, requires, among other things, a different conception of healing responsibilities. It requires a model in which the doctor assumes less than total responsibility for recovery and the patient assumes the power to aid his own healing.

External and Internal Physician. Medical science has made great advances during the last century. I remember a professor saying with obvious pride: "Ninety percent of all the scientists who have ever lived are alive today." Many of these scientists have discovered solutions for afflictions that have plagued man for thousands of years. Infectious diseases have been vastly reduced. Vaccines protect us from epidemics. Almost every day the newspapers report another life-saving achievement. In the light of this success, it is no wonder that the modern physician is often regarded with awe. His most elementary knowledge of pathology far surpasses anything the laymen could possibly know. Physicians assume and accept the power accorded to them. "When the president of a university confers honorary degrees on distinguished scholars his opening remarks are always the same: 'By virtue of the authority vested in me' . . . In much the same manner, our patients grant us the power to help them recover—not of course by royal decree or charter or a vote of the board, but rather by their need."[31] The assumption of authority and power is made by patient and physician alike.

Psychologically, however, the issue is more complex. The custom of relegating all healing responsibilities to the physician forces the adult patient to become a helpless child. A once healthy and dignified human being is no longer in charge of himself or his body. We have seen how comforting and stabilizing a childlike relationship can be for those with reliant personalities. But, once the intensity of a temporary regression has subsided, the extreme imbalance of healing responsibility inherent in our contemporary medical model can become self-defeating. This is especially true for those with strong, independent autonomous needs. The blunt split between the superior, all-knowing, responsible physician who "holds sickness and health in his hands" and the childlike, fearful, helpless patient can become an obstacle to recovery.

An "archetype" is an "inborn potentiality of behavior."[32] It is a typical universal response or image. The wise old man is an archetype that can be found in every culture. The eternal youth is another. The image of mother and child is yet another. These archetypes all have two poles, as does the one we are most interested in—a powerful image which has survived for thousands of years, the unitary image of the "healer-patient." There have always been sick people, there have always been healers (or physicians) and they have always formed an archetypal unit. We are patients when we become ill and seek a physician. But, since each of us possesses both poles of every archetype, including the "healer-patient," since there is a healer in every patient as well as a patient in every doctor, the union of patient-physician activates the corresponding force in each. The sick person relates himself to an external physician while simultaneously activating the healer within himself.[33]

The true physician heals others by knowing his own wounds as well as his medical text. He knows that if the inner healing factor is not engaged, the best medical attention in the world cannot cure his patient. Such statements as "He had no will to live" or "His inner resistance broke down" or "He didn't want to get well" all reflect the absence of an active inner healer. Spontaneous cures are rare (approximately one in ten thousand), but there are a vast number of patients who live comfortably with their cancers for many more years than is expected. These patients invariably have significant personal reasons for continuing life. Healing occurs when an alliance takes place between the physician's skills and the patient's inner healing potential. Those with reliant personalities achieve this alliance through great faith in their doctor. If the physician can inspire a positive attitude and a trust in the body's ability to recover, the inner healer has been actively engaged. Those with autonomous personalities usually approach their own capacity to heal more directly. They tend to assume an independent and conscious sphere of responsible activity. But there is an active inner healer at work whenever there is successful cancer treatment. No doctor, despite his vast knowledge, technology and skill, can achieve this success without the alliance with the patient's inner healer.

The Technique of Visualization. When the physician assumes total responsibility for the treatment of a patient and disregards the patient's attitude and healing potential, he loses a necessary ally and compromises the patient's recovery. When a patient rejects a physician and searches for a "miracle cure," he also loses a valuable ally and also splits the curative unit of the healer-patient archetype. There are now more physicians and a growing number of clinics which are beginning to offer a more holistic approach to cancer treatment. Institutions and traditions change slowly but they do undergo change. At present, the thrust of change is decidedly in the direction of greater respect for the needs of the patient and family. Health professionals have, once again, begun to consider the importance of emotion, attitude and the inner healer in treatment procedures.

Two of the pioneers in this area of cancer treatment are O. Carl Simonton, M.D., and his wife Stephanie Mathews-Simonton. Their clinic combines traditional medicine with a method of activating the patient's healing potential. No miracles are promised. They and others are trying to restore the symmetry of the healer-patient archetype by creating a true alliance between internal and external physician. I therefore want to present their work briefly, as an example of what is possible. The Simonton approach is a good illustration of what can be accomplished and of how a sense of personal authority can be brought into the process of cancer treatment.

Cancer patients who come to the Simonton Clinic for help must be under a physician's care and they must have already practiced the technique of visualization discussed below.* Patients, families and other important people in the patient's life, all of whom come with a "belief system" about cancer (cancer equals pain, suffering and death), are oriented toward the possibilities of recovery—the possibilities of mind, attitude and body. Patients receive individualized instruction in the technique of visualization. There are many names for this approach but they are all basically the same. The patient is taught how to relax and how to visualize his *cancer,* his *treatment* and his body's *immune mechanisms.* The relaxation and visualization are practiced three times a day. Patients and family members attend group sessions for five days in a residential retreat setting. These discussions deal with problems related to cancer, ways in which they can participate in the health process and goal setting, and visualization. Once the technique has been integrated, patients return home, and are monitored by their physicians.

To use visualization each patient creates a personal mental *picture* of his cancer, his treatment and his body's immune system. These images reveal a great deal about his attitudes toward the cancer and his body's ability to confront it. One man said his cancer looked "like a big black rat"; his treatment (chemotherapy) looked "like little

*Visualization and the Simonton approach to cancer are explained on a tape which can be obtained from the Cancer Counselling and Research Center, 1413 Eighth Avenue, Fort Worth, Texas 96104.

yellow pills." When asked what happened between the pills and the rat, he replied, "Once in a while the rat eats one of the pills . . . he's sick for a while but he always gets better and he bites me all the harder." When asked about his body's defense mechanisms, he said, "You know how eggs sit under the warm light? Well, they're incubating in there [his white blood cells] and one day they're going to hatch."[34] Patients who picture their cancer as big and powerful, who picture their treatment and immune systems as small and weak, are expecting ultimate destruction. They may well be able to confront the destructive process by modifying these images and expectations. It is possible to create and support a picture of one's white cells annihilating a defenseless cancer. One patient effected this change by visualizing hungry dogs who tore apart a cancer which resembled hamburger meat. By clarifying these images, the visualization technique provides some indication of how well the body defenses are functioning. It also provides a means of changing negative belief systems. The technique is to be practiced unvaryingly three times a day.

Biofeedback procedures have demonstrated astonishing degrees of mental influence over physically remote and microscopic body functions. Although this idea does not rest easily with our current concepts of medical treatment, the effectiveness of these procedures has been well documented. But do the visualization procedures work as well? It is too early to know for sure but the indications are encouraging. The first sixty patients treated by means of the Simonton visualization protocol (too small a number to be statistically meaningful, but important, nevertheless, since all the patients were considered "incurable" when they came for therapy) showed a remarkable trend.[35] The life expectancy for the group was nine months but they averaged two and a half times this statistical norm. Even more exciting is the fact that 70 percent of these sickest of all cancer patients returned to those activities in which they were engaged prior to the diagnosis of cancer. The quality of their lives shifted from that of helpless incurable patients to that of active human beings. These results are only an indication of what benefits might derive from a true partnership between external physician and internal healer. But the concepts are being applied and hopes are justifiably rising. The Simontons discuss their work and explain the protocol in their forthcoming book to be published by J. P. Tarcher Publications in 1978.

The technique of visualization is even more applicable to those who are not in terminal stages. I have worked with cancer patients who use the visualization technique faithfully. Most of these patients have either been in long remissions or have no evidence of cancer. Although it is impossible to know whether or not the absence of symptoms is directly related to the disciplined use of visualization, it is possible to attest unequivocally to its immense psychological value. The visualization technique offers a profound and effective activity to offset the role of victim. It provides a dramatic counteracting force to the image of relentless destructiveness so often associated with cancer. And it produces a dramatic reemergence of personal authority and self-esteem. Heart patients and diabetic patients retain a share of control by monitoring their diets, drugs and physical activities. Cancer patients can also acquire a sphere of active personal influence by practicing visualization procedures and psychologically monitoring their bodies' immune powers.

Some patients become ferociously defensive at the mere suggestion that there is a relationship between attitude and cancer. They seem to hear an unstated accusation that they are guilty of actively causing their cancers, or that they are to blame because their tumors have not vanished. Some patients are even berated by friends or family members who are overzealous partisans of the self-healing approach and who are as rigid in their thinking as are those physicians who dismiss all emotional influence. In certain settings, self-healing has become so fashionable that patients feel ashamed of their reliance on any form of traditional medicine. The shame is terribly misplaced. The exciting possibilities of exerting greater personal effectiveness and thereby enhancing cancer treatment are an important aspect of the active partnership with a physician. Awareness of one's inner healing potential provides an opportunity for sharing responsibility—not for assuming all of it. These new techniques introduce the possibility of influence; they offer a golden opportunity to assist the treatment process and they provide a means of reclaiming some areas of expanded personal authority. Continued tumor growth implies no moral or emotional failure. If each of us can approach the potential for inner healing with respect and perspective, we will have gained another area in which we can maintain our personal authority.

PART THREE

The Sphere of Family Influence

There is no major disease comparable to cancer in terms of its capacity to create emotional havoc within the family. But there are many ways in which an understanding of family dynamics can lead to the reduction of this stressful force.

To understand music, we must perceive it as more than a collection of individual notes. A melody emerges from their special relationships, from their rhythm and emphasis, from their harmonic or discordant alliances with one another. A family too is more than a group of individuals; to comprehend its essential form we must adopt this perspective of relationship. A family pattern emerges from the many currents that exist between its individual members; every family has a recognizable character and a distinctive tone. Its ethos is governed by subtle rules and reflected in specific family roles.

Four marriage patterns will be described. The same intense emotions of the cancer experience are reviewed from the perspective of family life. The impact of each experience varies with the areas of strength and vulnerability characteristic of each marriage pattern. These patterns or more precisely these "relationship tendencies" are capable of affording family members limitless opportunities for generosity and support. The patterns can also contain frustrating obstacles that are capable of escalating the stress of cancer treatment. Each of us can anticipate and avoid many of these predictable problems through an understanding of the structure of relationships.

7

The Structure of Relationship

And we are here as on a darkling plain
Swept with confused alarms of struggle and flight.
—MATTHEW ARNOLD

The image of cancer produces many of the same feelings in family members that it does in the cancer patient. In many instances, it is even more difficult for the parent, spouse or child of a cancer patient to manage the anxiety associated with the diagnosis and ensuing treatment of cancer. A major study of families with a child diagnosed and treated for leukemia showed that "only one family in ten emerged essentially intact . . . ninety per cent were seriously disrupted."[1] Cancer treatment evokes an enormous need for family stability. As one young wife and mother who had just completed her second major surgery for recurrent cancer described her need for familial support: "I feel surrounded by monsters of disease and despair. Ralph and those who love me are like an inner circle; they form a protective band around me. Without them I'd be dead."[2]

Unfortunately, in many instances, family bonds are so strained during the cancer crisis that bitter conflicts divide the family and augment the stress. The diagnosis and treatment of cancer are violent and unexpected blows to a family's sense of continuity and to their plans and dreams. Hopes and expectations can be so bitterly disappointed that the members of a family begin to blame one another for their fears, frustrations and pain. And yet, even under these difficult conditions, it is exceedingly rare for any of us to abandon our appeals for love and understanding. The following lines by Matthew Arnold were brought to me by one couple who said that the poem captured perfectly their sense of loss and despair, as well as their yearning:

> Ah, love, let us be true
> To one another! For the world, which seems
> To lie before us like a land of dreams,
> So various, so beautiful, so new,
> Hath really neither joy, nor love, nor light,
> Nor certitude, nor peace, nor help for pain;
> And we are here as on a darkling plain
> Swept with confused alarms of struggle and flight.

This couple could not understand how they had come into angry opposition when they wanted only to trust and support one another. They are not unique. There are too many families who experience themselves "swept with confused alarms," who experience neither "certitude, nor peace, nor help for pain," who despair of their loneliness and are bewildered by how it came to pass. And yet, with a measure of insight, courage, frankness and humor, the breakdown in familial relationships can be understood and avoided. Despite the grim realities of cancer, there is nothing dark and mysterious taking place within the family. Family members react to the cancer experience and to each other in a manner which can often be anticipated. With this knowledge and a willingness to assume new responsibilities, they can dramatically influence the effect cancer will have on their family life. They can, in fact, fulfill their desire to be "true to one another" and restore a great deal of light to their "darkling plain."

Moral Judgment and Pride

Members of a family affected by cancer are often reluctant to ascribe importance to their own feelings of stress. Many accuse themselves of being self-indulgent when they take care of their personal needs. Many believe that such behavior on their part indicates weakness of character or a selfishness of which they are terribly ashamed. Consequently, there is often a strong disinclination to admit that strain exists. Our pride may similarly make us reluctant to take family stress seriously and attend to its sources. Professional assistance may be experienced as intrusive "meddling" and rejected as irrelevant. It is as if each member of the family reasoned: "We have planned and argued, talked, learned and lived with each other for years. How could a stranger pretend to know us better than we know ourselves? How could a stranger, no matter how educated, offer worthwhile advice?"

The Value of Awareness

But the fact remains—the cancer crisis causes enormous stress within a family, and it is the way in which family members approach this stress that determines whether it will subside or grow to overwhelming proportions. All families are affected. When close and affectionate relationships exist, the stress may be felt as helplessness and frustration; patients experience themselves as terrible burdens to their families while family members despair of their inability to offer more effective help. If family relationships have been chronically strained, the stress will more likely lead to accusation and greater emotional distance.

Although all families are subject to cancer-related stress, no family is condemned to live out a burdensome existence. The preservation of family integrity may well require greater self-awareness and a willingness to be more forthright and flexible in one's behavior. Habitual modes of family life may well have to be altered, since family members can easily trap themselves in veiled but self-defeating rules that govern their behavior. And a broader perspective may be required or they may get caught in fixed roles that produce rigid patterns of interaction. Family patterns can be altered and individuals may become conscious of the roles they habitually play. I have

never worked with a family that did not have certain areas of una-
wareness which prevented family members from offering their full
support and love to one another. These "blind spots," until discovered, tend to absorb a great deal of emotional energy that is needed
for more important tasks during the cancer crisis.

The material presented in the following chapters will require a
willingness to consider down-to-earth family psychology. In order to
understand how the cancer experience affects a family, we must first
possess a basic understanding of how a family system works, of how
rules and roles regulate family life. Within the framework of this
understanding, I portray four relationship patterns and examine how
the cancer experience affects each of them. And finally I discuss the
way that patients and their families can avoid predictable pitfalls,
resolve areas of conflict, and establish, if they choose, cooperative
alliances during and following the siege imposed by cancer.[3]

The Family as a Working System

We begin with an illustration of a self-regulating system. The
human body maintains an average temperature of 98.6 degrees. In
winter or summer, on golf course or ski slope, the body's temperature remains between 97.3 and 99.1 degrees. The body compensates
for changes in the environment by means of complex regulating
mechanisms. In addition to involuntary systems such as perspiration
and capillary dilation, there are voluntary actions such as exercise
which also help to regulate our body temperature. If one mechanism
becomes impaired, other parts of the body's temperature-regulating
system will change in an attempt to compensate for the impairment.
The body has a sensing device, the skin, which is constantly sending
messages to the brain's control center to produce more heat or to
get rid of excess heat. If the body temperature rises above or falls
below its normal range, despite the efforts of its regulating mechanisms, then one of two important events is occurring. The temperature change might be a sign of body breakdown, of an *inability* to
maintain internal integrity. On the other hand, it might be a sign of

flexibility, of an *ability* to tolerate an unusual state of change for the purpose of survival, as when defending itself against infection.

A family also has regulating mechanisms, sensing abilities and tolerance levels. When a change occurs in a family, when a father loses his job, an older sister leaves home, or a mother becomes ill, the family members try to maintain their balance by means of compensatory changes. These attempts can be conscious and voluntary or they can occur in ways that are out of the family's awareness. For example, when a couple are emotionally estranged and in danger of separating, it may happen that one of their children becomes delinquent. The child and his parents are unaware that he is responding to a threatening change in the family. But his behavior may force his parents to deal with his problem and thereby keep them united in efforts to help him. In many instances, the delinquent child of parents threatened by divorce is the most desperately concerned with the family's impending rupture. His intense fear may be covered with a thin veneer of toughness or with a guilty denial of his concern. But he is the one who, knowingly or unknowingly, takes on the responsibility of trying to save the family balance.

The above description is an example of a process in which a family member behaves in a manner determined by the overall need of the family. His behavior is part of a regulating system.

We can see such regulating mechanisms at work in a son's reluctance to go to school when he sees how lonely his mom has become since dad began going on long business trips. We can also see them at work in a son's assumption of dad's family responsibilities after dad becomes withdrawn following his cancer treatment.

The family system can be more subtle but just as predictable with regard to unexpressed emotion.

> We lost a child to cancer five years ago . . . my husband and I are both people who tend to keep our feelings to ourselves, and we haven't even talked much about our little boy, since his death. . . . [But] we do have a rather unusual problem as our boy was an identical twin. Even though his brother was not three years old at the time, and as I said, we have not discussed it unduly, we have had some problems with his adjustment. Even after this length of time, he talks about his brother quite a lot, wishes

he were with us, and twice has said he ought to go out and "get run over" so he could "be in heaven with Jeffrey.". . . He walks and talks in his sleep, sometimes crying out and yelling and it is hard to get him calmed down.[4]

This eight-year-old is trying to express his family's secret grief; he is trying to heal the family's wound in the absence of any acknowledged sadness on the part of his parents. He is not aware of his job as "the family mourner," but he nevertheless performs his role of expressing the family's grief and pain.

From these examples we see how the family system attempts to compensate for change just as the body attempts to maintain its constant temperature. As with the body, these attempts can succeed or fail. If change or loss occurs, the family's tolerance is tested, and their fate often depends on their system's degree of flexibility. A body that can tolerate 105 degrees is a body that can fight off infection and survive. A family that can tolerate changes in their relationship patterns during the siege of cancer can also survive intact. But there is more. The family, like any living system, can do more than maintain itself. It can grow and change; the tiny newborn son who barely fills his cradle becomes the grown man who lifts you in his arms. When they are functioning well, family systems provide a balanced continuity for growth as well as for survival.

Family Roles and Family Rules

Systems of interaction develop by means of social roles. Our culture usually demands strength, decisive action and dependability in men; nurturance, emotion and dependence in women. These sexual roles often persist despite the dramatic successes of the women's movement. The *husband* of a convalescent wife must concern himself with the needs of children and with matters of school, meals, clothing and discipline. No matter how great his understanding of the situation, he will usually experience great strain when performing these unfamiliar tasks. The *father* of a seriously ill child, by social custom, is not permitted the same freedom of emotional expression as his wife. He is expected to be "strong" and is thereby deprived of the privilege of being emotional. Similar cultural restraints apply to women. There are, in fact, a multitude of special roles required within each family.

In this respect we may liken the complex uniqueness of human beings to dreams. Whether we recall them or not, studies have shown that we create an endless variety of images and unique stories every night. The mind is fathomless; our dreams display an infinite variety of forms, ideas and feelings. But recurrent nightmares can interrupt this natural flow. The same themes and images can plague us with stubborn and unchanging consistency. Such nightmares resemble family roles that have become overly rigid. They trap one area of our personality and, like a nightmare or a broken record, keep replaying the same theme over and over again. We get to know the theme well, others learn what to expect, there is security in the familiar patterns. But the burdens and limitations are obvious.

Family Integrity and Cancer-Related Stress

Family roles often provide needed comfort and stability during the cancer crisis. However, if they are not flexible and capable of shifting with the unprecedented demands of the cancer experience, they can also become primary obstacles to the successful management of stress. When a family member is hospitalized, unable to perform usual tasks or threatened by death, family rules often need to be revised and family roles often need to be modified. The family system attempts to find a new balance and these changes can evoke considerable anxiety.

Donald[5] was the dominant head of his family when he began cancer treatment. His wife, Jane, had always depended on his decisiveness and deferred to his preferences. Their fourteen-year-old son was a quiet, studious boy. During Donald's protracted treatment, he became progressively irritable, withdrawn, preoccupied and ultimately dependent on his wife. Jane was faced with the choice of asserting herself and assuming much more independence or of finding someone else to depend on. Unfortunately, she was unwilling to experience the anxiety and uncertainty of a new role and began turning helplessly to her son. He tried to take his dad's place by supporting his emotionally distraught mother but became depressed and began getting into trouble at school. Donald and Jane grew more depressed and finally sought professional counseling.

Donald's physical illness and treatment required role changes within the family that each would not tolerate. Donald could not bear to be dependent on his wife and became irritable and withdrawn. Jane could not tolerate unfamiliar responsibilities, and their son experienced too much conflict to compensate for all the family changes. Donald recovered and the family balance was partially restored. But the major stress experienced by each of them could have been prevented. Their difficulties arose from the vulnerability of their family system, their lack of understanding and their inflexibility, much more than it did from Donald's cancer treatment.

Despite the specific roles we play, most families experience stormy times of stress and most families know quiet periods of easy harmony. There are no patterns guaranteed to eliminate the stress inherent in life, and we know of none that can prevent all of the anxieties and fears associated with cancer treatment. Fortunately marriage is not reserved for the "stable, spartan, tee-totaler, blessed with private income, born of atypically diplomatic parents, attached to church, conservative in investments, possessed of true standards, gleefully sexual and of Solomonic wisdom."[6] As less than perfect human beings, we create our unique family relationships and evolve our unique family ethos, but there is a rhythm and reason to the shifting moods of our lives and to the roles we create. As we accommodate ourselves to one another and develop ways to get along and satisfy mutual needs, we establish recognizable patterns of relationship. These prevailing modes of interaction are rarely perceived by individual members of a family but are easily experienced by a sensitive visitor. It is the influence of these unrecognized but pervasive patterns that all too often determines the outcome of the cancer crisis.

Typical Marital Tendencies

In the following chapters we will examine four common patterns of interaction; they have been selected because they provide important insights into many of the stressful marital conflicts associated with the cancer crisis. These four relationship tendencies appear most frequently in my clinical practice.[7] The two "complementary" patterns are characterized by *differences* in the marriage partners (opposites attracting); the two "symmetrical" ones by *similarities* in the partners (like attracting like). Some experts[8] argue that men and women are first drawn to one another by their shared values, interests and backgrounds, but that they remain interested in one another because of differences in their personalities. The reality may be more complex. There are those of us who look for the contrast and complement to ourselves: a playful presence to complement stiff formality, a childlike dependence to complement parental authority, a lusty passion to complement sexual inhibition. Others seek a mirror image of themselves: a kind and peaceful demeanor, an intellectual preoccupation, a robust and challenging manner, a minimal appetite for life, all reminiscent of themselves. Those who seek a complement hope for a relationship that will enlarge their range of experience. Those who search for symmetry seek fulfillment through what is known and valued.

There is an almost infinite variety and uniqueness in our experience of one another. And yet this complex diversity may be profitably examined from the viewpoint of general tendencies and shared patterns. It is my purpose to describe some of those predictable themes which emerge when human beings form relationships with one another. The discussion that follows is not intended as a literal description of any given relationship. Dramatic illustrations have been used to make the proposed patterns as vivid and understandable as possible. While they may at times appear extreme, everything discussed in these chapters is a part of normal family life. Since we are concerned with preventing the breakdown of relationships, I have focused attention primarily on the vulnerable areas of each pattern. Those tendencies which may evoke delight, reassurance and respect, but do not present apparent problems to family members, I have touched upon in passing but have not lingered over. It is my intention to examine those delicate areas of potential conflict which make life so difficult for patients and their families during the cancer crisis. And it is my hope that, by growing familiar with those areas in which conflicts typically arise, we may develop sufficient understanding to avoid and resolve them.

8

The Hare-Tortoise Marriage Pattern

It is nothing new indeed that generous young persons
often admire most what nature hasn't given them.
—HENRY JAMES, *The Wings of the Dove*

The Fable

A couple with a leukemic child reported[1] the following marital
impasse:

BARBARA: ... from the time we found out, Joe has closed up like a
clam. He offers no support, won't talk about Karen's illness, says I'm
too emotional. ... It tears me up. I know how bad he feels, I know
how sad he is but he's so damn uninvolved. I feel so alone and it tears
me to pieces. ...

JOE: She's at me all the time and she never stops asking me for something. I need to be left alone. She doesn't understand how much I have
to do. I don't have all the answers, and crying isn't going to help me
get them. ... I'm trying to do everything possible and she is just about
driving me crazy.

Over a period of two years an angry tension between Joe and Barbara had replaced the sympathies they usually felt for one another.
Their grievances are so typical and so recognizable that they provide
us with an excellent starting point. Let us consider what is taking

place below the surface of these common complaints by exploring their responses to a familiar story. In one interview I asked Joe and Barbara if they knew the fable of the Tortoise and the Hare.

> JOE: I always hated that story. That slow, dumb turtle plodding along in a rut. Who wants to win a race if that's the way you have to go through life.
>
> BARBARA: (embarrassed and laughing at the strength of his response): Really, I've always hated the ridiculous, scatter-brained rabbit. He can never finish anything and only runs around in a stupid frenzy.

This is the fable: A vivacious, provocative Hare constantly teased a quiet, dependable Tortoise about his slow, careful pace. The Tortoise retaliated by challenging the Hare to a race. In a flash the Hare was off, racing far ahead of the deliberate, steady Tortoise, who plodded along in his usual unhurried way. After a while, the Hare stopped to wait for the Tortoise. He rested in the sun and fell asleep. The Tortoise plodded on, passed the sleeping Hare and crossed the finish line just as the Hare awoke with an embarrassed start. The moral: Slow and steady wins the race.

Barbara and Joe are highly critical of the *emotional tendencies* which they recognize with great discomfort in the animals of this fable. It was, however, these same emotional temperaments which first drew them together and then led to their painful estrangement during Karen's illness. Let us examine how this might have happened.

Hare-Tortoise Relationship Characteristics

A man and a woman[2] predisposed to a Hare-Tortoise relationship pattern are unknowingly seeking for what they feel to be lacking in themselves. He is irresistibly drawn to her enthusiasm, vivaciousness and warm spontaneity, attracted by her life force, by her ability to have fun and by the way she seems so effortlessly capable of intimacy. Inside, he is insecure, unable to feel fully alive and awkward at initiating emotional closeness. He hopes that she will bring a sparkle of life into his blander emotional existence, that she will provide him with an experience of close human contact.

She is just as irresistibly drawn to his steadiness and his ability to be logical, organized and reassuringly dependable. She also is insecure and often confused by her intense and varied experiences. She is sometimes in doubt about her desirability and hopes that he will bring to her a feeling of protection and safety.

Each seeks in the other that which he suspects to be deficient in himself and each hopes to achieve wholeness by means of what the other brings into the relationship. Henry James has described just such a couple: ". . . any deep harmony that might eventually govern them would not be the result of their having much in common—having anything, in fact, but their affection; and would really find its explanation, in some sense, on the part of each, of being poor where the other was rich. It is nothing new indeed that generous young persons often admire most what nature hasn't given them."[3]

But the problems begin when each discovers that the other is not the ideally imagined spouse and each experiences a certain amount of disappointment and resentment. It is of special interest to us that, during periods of confrontation, the very qualities which were originally attractive and filled with so much promise are experienced in predictably different ways. During a bitter disagreement, he is no longer seen as a good, stable, dependable, silent man, but is perceived as a closed, disapproving, insensitive, uninvolved "clam." She is no longer seen as a vivacious, spontaneous, warm woman, but experienced as an irrational, overreactive, blaming, hysterical "shrew."

Shortly after I began to meet with Joe and Barbara, I asked them each to illustrate graphically a typical moment of frustration, to make a family sculpture of their experience of the marriage at that time. Barbara had Joe sink into his chair and look away with a stubborn unseeing stare. She stood behind him and said she felt "unimportant, ignored and separate." He placed her standing before him, a look of critical reproach on her face and an accusing finger directed at his nose. He said he felt "like running away from her constant accusations."

The manner in which the Hare-Tortoise couple fight is reflected in these family sculptures and is determined largely by their respective areas of vulnerability. He suffers from a nagging sense of self-doubt and therefore needs a great deal of approval, appreciation and muted admiration. He needs to be seen and to experience himself as a "good" man who is "right" about things. Because of this self-doubt and the accompanying fear of being exposed, he can be easily wounded by her pointed accusations. She, on the other hand, suffers from a nagging fear of being rejected and needs constant reassurance of his emotional presence. Because of this fear of abandonment, his silent, stubborn withdrawal fills her with alarm and anxiety.

The Hare-Tortoise couple typically struggle in the following manner: An issue will arise. He will withdraw and become emotionally less accessible. She will become anxious, try to draw him out, and if unsuccessful begin to taunt him or let him know he is behaving badly. Since, in these situations, she usually has greater verbal agility and a gift for striking some area of his insecurity, he begins to feel more and more exposed and inept. He will often respond with an even more angry withdrawal. Rather than experience his growing sense of ineptitude and resentment, he soothes his hurt feelings by persuading himself that he acts according to noble motives. He might say to himself: "This is outrageously unfair! I'm a good man and I'm trying to act in a responsible and reasonable manner while she is being hysterical and unreasonably abusive. I'll silently suffer her accusations until she sees that I'm right."

She perceives his "silent suffering" as indifference, disapproval and rejection and therefore becomes even more resourceful in attempting to break through his shell. She is quite aware of her abusive style and might justify it by saying to herself, "I'm being nasty, that's true, but he has no right to run away. There is a real problem to be dealt with and since he's disappeared into his shell, it's up to me to force him out and make him face facts. If I act in an extreme manner, it's only because *I'm really concerned* and besides, it's his fault."

The struggle will continue until either she is no longer able to stand his withdrawal or he can no longer stand her attacks on his integrity. One familiar ending to the struggle follows her change in tactics: she dissolves into tears or childish helplessness; he is then free to come forward and comfort her. In this way, the familiar pattern —he providing the steady, reliable comfort and she providing emotion and intimacy—is reestablished.

But let's look a little more closely at the way they fight. Although each can wound the other and invariably chooses the most vulnerable place to attack, they do so with differing amounts of awareness. Her accusations are open and direct. She might ennoble the reasons for her behavior, but will readily admit to being frustrated and angry. On the other hand, he is often unaware of what he feels and how he fights. Although he justifies his withdrawal as an attempt to be "reasonable" and "good," his behavior is as much a fighting strategy as is her direct assault. Since he has the greater tolerance for tension, his tactic of withdrawal is often the more effective. However, in order to be effective, he must deceive himself into believing that he is not fighting; he must remain oblivious of the most obvious consequences of his angry behavior and insist on being taken at face value. But his "innocent" silence can be extremely cruel, for it says, "I'm shutting you out. I'm punishing you by withholding my thoughts and feelings."

In summary, the Hare-Tortoise couple are a *complementary* pair who tend to fight in a typical manner when they are angry, frightened or hurt. She is overt, explosive and assaultive; her strategy is to "blame and shame" him. And since he is vulnerable to assaults upon his sense of being "good" and "right," her blaming strategies can be extremely effective. He is covert, implosive and withdrawn; his strategy is to "retreat and shame" her. Since she is dependent and often ashamed of behaving like a "shrew," his withdrawal intensifies her shame and is thereby also extremely effective. Although these dynamics are often as flagrant as described above, they more often assert themselves in less dramatic form. By glance and gesture, by muted, indirect conversation, an atmosphere is created in which the Hare-Tortoise tendencies may occur outside the awareness of the participants and thereby become the more binding upon them.

The Hare-Tortoise Pattern and Cancer-Related Stress

Three of the most common sources of anxiety associated with the image of cancer cause particular distress to those who relate in the Hare-Tortoise manner. The sense of losing control over one's life, the fear of being abandoned and the image of a hidden, sinister "shadow" force are all important aspects of the cancer experience. They all strike particularly vulnerable areas of the Hare-Tortoise relationship pattern.

Temperament and Loss of Control. The wife in the Hare-Tortoise couple needs to be able to depend on a steady, logical and confident man since she often experiences herself as "too emotional" and "too irrational." How vulnerable she therefore is to the devastating sense of irrationality that accompanies the diagnosis of cancer. The image of her emotions raging out of control is one of her greatest personal sources of anxiety, and it is concretely represented in the form of cancer. A cancer patient says: "I just don't know where to turn. Everything is just too much for me."[4] The mother of a child being treated for cancer says: "I'm drowning in all my feelings. I run around in circles and sometimes I'm really nasty. I just can't help myself."[5]

The anxiety aroused by the loss of control characteristic of cancer is just as great for her husband. The father of a child being treated for cancer says: "I've got to pull myself together. Joan [his wife] is going in all directions so I must stay strong . . . crying is just going to upset him. . . . Kent must have confidence in me. I can't waste any time sobbing with her. I've got to hold on and stay together for Kent's sake."[6] In an effort to deal with the terrifying unknowns and loss of control associated with cancer, this father responds in a predictable way; he pulls into an emotional shell and tries to organize his thoughts and feelings.

Although each of them is susceptible to that part of the cancer experience that involves a sense of losing control, they respond in very different ways. The following is another example of these differing responses. The wife of a cancer patient says: "He won't tell me anything. He keeps all these secrets about the business, about our stocks. It's important that I know these things but he's so evasive." Her husband replies, "I'm putting things in order. I need some time to do it. Some quiet time without a lot of hassle. Everything will be okay, just give me some space."[7] Each feels alarm and loss of control; each describes the experience of "everything slipping away." But their temperamental differences lead to conflict. He needs to withdraw and organize his affairs, she needs to get them opened up, discussed and understood.

The Hare-Tortoise partners differ in their self-appointed areas of responsibility with regard to this loss of control. In most situations, he assumes the responsibility of keeping order, of being logical and of solving problems. But he cannot solve the problem of cancer and he turns exclusively to those practical areas that afford him some degree of control and competence, some possibility of "doing something." This attempt to deal with his anxiety also leads to marital problems in the Hare-Tortoise relationship. The father of a child being treated for cancer says: "I'm doing everything I can think of to make things all right, but she doesn't understand. Nothing is ever enough for her."[8] The mother of the same child replies, "Most of the problems don't have easy answers and I get no support from him. I give all the time and never get a breather. [*What makes you cry just now?*] I feel so sad and frustrated, he just won't see what's going on. He makes me feel weak because I want to talk."

The following is another typical example of the same relationship pattern and the ease with which such partners can misunderstand one another. It is typical because, once again, the husband burdens himself with the misguided expectation that he must do something to solve the problem. The husband of a woman caring for her terminally ill mother explains: "She's very upset, it's hard for her. She was really close to her mother. . . . I tell her don't talk to me, I'm no psychiatrist. [*How do you feel when she talks about her sadness?*] I feel lousy. I'm sorry for her but I don't know what to do. Damn, I can't cure her mother."[9] By assuming that she only wanted him to *do something* and defending himself against his inability to do anything concrete, he became unable to hear her appeal for something even more important. "You won't understand. I don't want you to cure her, or to do anything like that. I feel so awful. I can't take any more pressure. I don't want a psychiatrist. All I want is you to help me a little; all I want is one comforting place to come home to. I feel so sad and you make me so angry. Why can't you just listen?"

The wife in the Hare-Tortoise couple does not have her husband's capacity to "push aside" intense emotions. They grow, continue to oppress her and threaten to break out of control. Far from being reassured by his unwillingness to show his feelings or by his preoccupation with practical, unemotional necessities, she begins to fear that she will "tear to pieces inside." In this manner, the sense of losing control that almost always attends the diagnosis of cancer tragically dovetails with one of the most difficult areas of this couple's relationship. When anxiety becomes too oppressive, she will begin to blame him for being uninvolved and irresponsible and he will begin to blame her for being too emotional and weak. Both are desperately struggling with their experience of losing control in their own distinctive way and both tend to misunderstand the attempts of the other.

The Hare and Rejection. Dependency and underlying fear of rejection give rise to much of the wife's behavior in the Hare-Tortoise relationship. The universal fear of abandonment associated with cancer cannot help but trigger her underlying chronic fear of rejection. In the following instance,[10] a wife finally begins to confront her withdrawn and moody husband seven months following *his* successful cancer treatment. Their fourteen-year-old daughter, Lilian, and sixteen-year-old daughter, Nancy, are also present.

JUDY (MOTHER):   He just wants to be left alone and I'm sick of it. You had cancer, that's true, but you want us to do all the adjusting, you won't do any and I'm just sick of it. If you want so much distance, why don't you physically remove yourself? It's just a pretense to sit here and say we have a marriage and a family. You're not involved and you don't want to be. [Long silence. I say to George, *What is this touching in you?*]

GEORGE (FATHER):   It doesn't touch me, she's so removed from understanding even a millionth of what I have to face. What might be valid for her is completely canceled out by her lack of understanding. I'm in another frame of mind and you all have to face it whether you like it or not. If you had gone through this you'd understand why I want to be left alone. [*Would you like them to understand what you're going through?*] . . . It doesn't matter. [*Does it matter that Judy is so angry she's asking you to change or leave?*] . . . I'm not the same person I was before my surgery. I don't pretend to be. I'm more closed. . . .

JUDY: I feel used and I hate the way you push me away. That's 90 percent of it. I can't live this way any more. [*Can you tell George what's so difficult for you?*] You're saying you're going in some separate direction, maybe it's a direction I'm not included in.

GEORGE: That's not true.

JUDY: But you have all the controls. I see your needs but how far do I have to go with something I don't feel myself capable of doing. You announce that you need to be left alone in such a superior sense, like all of us are groveling down here while you're the superior person up there.

GEORGE: I've no answer to that kind of stuff. [To fourteen-year-old Lilian—*You keep looking at mom and frowning. What do you want to say to her?*]

LILIAN (VERY SOFTLY):   You're so hard on him. You really are. He's been sick, how can you keep saying things like that?

JUDY (HARSHLY):   'Cause I'm a cold, hard bitch and you shut up!

LILIAN: But, ma, all he's saying is to please leave him alone and you're on him all the time.

JUDY (CRYING AND THEN COLDLY SILENT, AND THEN):   No one can say anything to their father so they take it out on me. Since his surgery they are afraid to say anything that's not nice to him. So here it is, "Oh, mom, what are you doing to dad, poor dad." How about what dad is doing to us? [To Lilian and Nancy—*Do you feel mom's the villain here?*]

LILIAN: No, but . . . [*But what? Tell mom.*] I'm so scared you're going to force dad to leave us. (Begins to weep. Long pause.)

NANCY (SIXTEEN-YEAR OLD):   I keep getting the feeling that he's trying to make us get along without him, trying to wean us, like he's not going to be here for very long.

GEORGE: How old are you?

NANCY: Dad, you know how old I am . . . isn't it time you leveled with us?

GEORGE (QUIETLY):   You're still too young to understand certain things. [*What is your fantasy, Nancy, about dad?*]

NANCY: I don't know. [*What do you imagine Dad is thinking and feeling?*] Maybe he's shutting us out to prepare us.
GEORGE: That's ridiculous, of course not.
NANCY (BITTERLY): Well, I don't know that . . .

There are many things taking place in this conversation. But Lilian and Nancy, like their mother, all share the same alarm: they fear being abandoned. Judy responds with anger: "I hate the way you push me away." Her daughter Lilian responds with open fear and blame: "I'm so scared you're going to force dad to leave us." The older daughter Nancy responds with speculation: "Maybe he's shutting us out to prepare us." Emotional withdrawal, as we see it here with George, will inevitably evoke the fear of being rejected, since a partial emotional abandonment has already occurred. The wife in a Hare-Tortoise relationship pattern is particularly vulnerable to this experience. Yet it is difficult for both of them to realize that it was not the cancer but their behavior that was responsible for the experience of agitated aloneness.

What is it, however, that would lead a husband with so much motivation toward being a "good man" to act in such a stubborn manner? A large part of his withdrawal is a response to another specific aspect of his experience of cancer.

The Tortoise and the Shadow Side. Since the self-esteem of the husband in the Hare-Tortoise relationship depends in large measure on his sense of being a "good man" who conducts himself with quiet integrity, his ideal qualities are antithetical to those associated with the image of cancer. He clings to an image of himself as effective, dependable, knowledgeable, organized and kind, but the diagnosis of cancer penetrates the boundaries of his being with an image of sinister force, evil excess, recklessness, destructiveness and uncontrollable greed. The image of cancer evokes our "shadow side" and the husband in this relationship pattern is now faced with a disease which represents aspects of himself long denied. Any experience that makes him question his sense of being good, right and dependable is extremely painful and disconcerting to him. His distress and shame often lead to withdrawal and compensatory statements that make his wife feel ashamed or in some way responsible for his distress.

George says: "Everything was fine until my surgery. It's been really hard. I need some understanding but she's cold and bitchy and won't even have sex. She's taken my courage and my sense of responsibility away. I just need her to be nice. She should do that, it's not asking too much."

With cancer-related stress, he is particularly vulnerable and in need of support from Judy. He is less armored than usual and therefore easily wounded by any remarks that point to his deficiencies. At a time when he is withdrawn, struggling with these dark forces and in particular need of approval and appreciation, his spouse out of anxiety and self-defense is often blaming him for being inadequate. Judy replies: "I'm a bitch, I know. I push and push to provoke him into being a man, not a whipped dog; he's like a pathetic little boy following me around. I can't stand it. I need a shoulder to lean on. I want to scream when someone says, 'You're so strong.' I'm not, damnit, I'm just human. He either brings me cookies like I'm a little girl or begs for sympathy like I'm his mom. I don't want to be anywhere near him."

It is not surprising that those in Hare-Tortoise relationships tend to attack one another. The cancer experience has evoked the deepest fears in each of them and has forced them to experience the least-comforting aspects of their particular relationship. What, then, can they do?

Resolving the Hare-Tortoise Marital Impasse

The Hare-Tortoise couple are distinguished primarily by the way in which they differ from one another. Since their relationship is a complementary one, their greatest strength and opportunity may well be inherent in these differences. Their capacity to tolerate, accept and profit from the manifest ways in which they are different will determine the course of their marriage during the enormous stress unleashed by the diagnosis of cancer and can provide the primary means by which the Hare-Tortoise couple may maintain and deepen their capacity to comfort one another.

Let us exploit two cultural stereotypes in order to make a useful analogy and enlarge this perspective of *difference*. Imagine, for a moment, an Irish wake. Picture a group of mourners consoling each other by allowing themselves open license for great emotional release, exuberantly expressing their intense feelings, be they of sorrow or festive celebration, as a means of dealing with a death and a loss. Now imagine an English country funeral—quiet, somber, unemotional, politely restrained and monumentally dignified; a group of mourners comforting one another by containing their intense feelings, by controlling any expression of strong emotion and by doing what is expected of them.

These two cultural clichés serve us well, for they echo the Hare-Tortoise temperaments. The Irish mourners share many of the qualities of the wife, especially her need to talk and express feelings as the primary way in which she deals with intense emotion. The English mourners resemble her husband, particularly his need to contain and control his feelings. When the husband demands that his wife adopt his approach to the stress of cancer, he is asking her to give up *her* basic means of coping. His demand resembles a self-righteous Englishman marching into the middle of an Irish wake and insisting that everyone "stop all the nonsense, be strong and keep a stiff upper lip." When the wife coercively pushes her husband into her approach, she is likewise stripping him of *his* basic means of coping with cancer, and her demands resemble a self-righteous Irishman storming into a staid English reception and raucously berating them all to "let themselves go."

The Irish mourner, when faced with intense emotion, chooses to go inside it, to experience it until the emotion subsides or is resolved. The English mourner, when faced with similar intense emotion, tends to marshal defensive forces against it until the intense feeling seems defeated and once again under control. Cancer-related experiences of anxiety and depression can be formidable indeed. In the Hare-Tortoise relationship, an "Irish mourner" and an "English mourner" are married to one another. When they experience the impact of cancer, their approach, their temperamental choice of confrontation will be fundamentally and predictably different.

When this couple face the stress of cancer, she needs to experience and express her feelings, he needs to contain and control his. If each can understand that the approach of the other is not wrong but simply different, is another and equally valid way of dealing with anxiety, then the first important step toward a supportive alliance will have taken place.

The following poignant example portrays a woman who instinctively chose the Hare approach to the pain of an inoperable tumor:

> A young woman at our hospital refused any narcotic that dulled her awareness. Although she was often in great pain, she desperately wanted her senses and her experiences to be clear. One day I asked her how she dealt with her pain and she replied, "How do *you* deal with waves when you are swimming in the ocean?" I told her I ducked under them and she said, "It's the same. If you fight the waves, they knock you over. If you try to outswim them, they catch you. But if you go under them, they break over you with much less impact. This is exactly what I do with my waves of pain. But I'm frightened! The waves of pain are getting larger and there is very little water left to go down under. It's shallow and sandy. What will I do if there's no water left and I can't get under the pain?" About a week later we talked again and I asked about her pain. "I now know what to do," she replied. "I realized I was still fighting by trying to go under it. Now I've really let go. I'm a part of the wave, a part of the water and of the sand. I'm mixing with all of them. The sea is taking me back and I feel so peaceful."[11]

This woman, by her insistence on surrendering to her pain, had a rare experience, an experience that included a degree of suffering few of us would be willing to go through, but one in which the transcendence of pain was ultimately accomplished. It is clear that a person with a Hare approach, even when the tendency and the circumstances are much less extreme, needs to be aware of what she is experiencing. To have given this woman morphine against her will would have sabotaged her unique temperament and robbed her of one of the most meaningful experiences of her entire life. The husband of such a woman, if they share a Hare-Tortoise relationship pattern, would want her to be out of pain and he would be tempted to insist that she be given a pain-killing narcotic. It would be his task, therefore, to understand how different her temperament is from his own, to respect that difference by not imposing his approach, and to offer her all the generosity of which he is capable.

The Appreciation of Difference. Marilyn[12] was extremely involved in her mother's cancer treatment. She described herself as her mother's "best friend." Marilyn's fear and anxiety were extreme, but no more extreme than her need for sympathetic support by her much less emotional and much less involved husband, who said he could not stand any more of her intense moods. She tried to explain herself to him: "I keep thinking of that book about crossing the ocean on a raft, you know, that RA expedition, I think. Remember, we talked about it. The papyrus reeds bent and stretched with the swaying of the sea but the oak oars and the oak rudder broke with the first storm. The reed boat made it across the ocean, but the strong wood couldn't help at all . . . at first I tried to be like you, like the oak rudder, and I felt like I would break in two. Now when I begin to feel a storm inside, I try to bend like the reeds of that boat." Her husband shook his head, understanding but not wanting to understand. Finally, he smiled at her and said, "I'll bend with you as much as this old trunk of mine will let me." That he understood what she was experiencing and acknowledged the validity of her temperamental choice was all she really needed from him. In fact, he didn't have to bend at all; he had only to stay with her as she crossed *her* stormy sea.

The Hare-Tortoise relationship, if left to itself, can strain to the breaking point during the stress of the cancer experience. She tends to become more abusive and more intrusive as he tends to become more withdrawn and armored. As each grows more mistrustful, disappointed and resentful, a competitive "sit down strike" can develop. This impasse occurs when they settle into stubbornness. However, even when emotionally depleted, there are always areas in which each can be generous and still maintain his or her integrity. Bob and Joann[13] were struggling at such an impasse. His mother, who had lived with them for many years, was dying of inoperable cancer. Let us listen to a part of their angry conversation:

BOB: Look, I'm under enough pressure already. It's a lousy time for you to be screaming about your feelings.

JOANN: Of course it's lousy, that's why I'm screaming. This is the time I'm feeling all these things, for you, for your mother. . . . I'm angry, I'm sad, and see, right now you're closing off again. All you can think about is yourself, you won't deal with anything.

BOB: Look, just please don't bother me any more. This is the worst time in the world for you to be playing these emotional games. [*Can you tell Bob what you're experiencing at this moment?*]

JOANN: I'm hurt and furious. I don't want to ask you for anything. I don't give a damn what happens. I've been burned so much, shut out so many times, that I just want to hurt you back. [*Bob, what do you see in Joann's face right now?*]

BOB: She seems very upset, sad, almost at her wit's end. [*What do you imagine she's so upset about?*] About me, of course. She wants me to do things. But what more am I supposed to do? Tell the doctors how to treat my mother? Just what else am I supposed to do?

JOANN (QUIETLY):   Let yourself feel something.

BOB: It's perfectly clear, I feel very bad.

JOANN (LOUDER):   There must be more. It's natural, it's normal, it just is, for God's sake.

BOB (ALMOST WHINING):   Why? Why the hell must there be more?

JOANN (SCREAMING):   Because there just is! (Long pause.) [*Joann, if you were Bob, what would you be feeling these days?*] I'd be angry, she's just lying there in the hospital and she's dying and there's nothing I can do. I'd feel lost and frightened, too. She's so dear and she's dying and I'd be very sad. [*And if you were Bob, how would you handle such feelings?*] I'd want to be alone, I'd get off by myself. [*Why?*] Because I'd be confused and hurt and I wouldn't quite know what to say or what to do. [*And how could Joann help?*] By being warm and letting me do the things I can do without demanding a lot more right now. [*Check with Bob and see if what you imagine is true.*]

BOB: Exactly. I feel bad and need some peace. [*And now you, Bob, make believe you're Joann for a moment, try to imagine that you're in her shoes. Now as Joann you understand how Bob feels, so what makes you keep bothering him?*] Because it isn't fair. He does so little and I'm stuck with everything, the kids, all the arrangements, telling everyone what's happening, and I'm not getting any help. And I'd be jealous. I love his mom, too, but she only asks about him. It's just not fair that he always leaves me in such a stew. [*What are you most angry at him for?*] For not doing anything to help me when he knows how much I need him to, right now. For being so selfish and weak. [*How is he selfish?*] It would be so easy to just spend some time together, to be concerned with me and how I was doing. And it wouldn't kill him to be a little more open. [*Ask Joann how accurate these assumptions about what she's feeling and thinking are.*]

JOANN: I don't think you're weak, but the rest is true. [*What is especially true for you?*] That I feel deserted and stuck with everything. [*Are you surprised that Bob understands?*] Sort of; I usually think he just sees me as a nagging bitch.

Bob and Joann could imagine what the other was experiencing and they continued to talk about their worst fears and their mutual mistrust, about how they were preventing themselves from being as generous as in the past and how much they wanted to trust each other once again. In this instance, Bob slowly came to understand that he could let Joann into his private world without being over-whelmed by her intense emotions and needs. He began to trust her ability to respect his temperament and his personal boundary. Joann began to give him more privacy as she began to trust his willingness to initiate contact with her and as she came to see his acknowledg-ment of the validity of her emotions. The changes came about slowly, by trial and error and with periodic setbacks. One time he attempted to reassure her: "I read an article once about how mourn-ing for some people has to be a totally private process. It's true for me and I'm already beginning to grieve for mom and for myself too. When I see how upset you are, I want to go as far away from you as I can. I can't handle everything at once. . . . It's not you I want to get away from, it's what you're feeling." This was the first time she had heard him say that he was feeling any grief at all and she asked him to tell her this again. He continued repeating that he was "sad and needed to be alone with his feelings" and this obvious message, frequently heard, made it possible for her to say, "When I know he is grieving, I can convince myself that he is all right and then I can leave him alone."

In these two instances, each individual was able to respect and accept his or her own temperamental need. Having accepted themselves, each was then able to be generous to the other. And, by accepting their differences, each found a way to be sensitive to the other's need without sacrificing his or her sense of integrity. Marilyn accepted her need to "bend" like the reeds of a papyrus raft, and her husband was able to acknowledge that need. His recognition of *her temperamental preference* allowed him to comfort her rather than to defend himself; to be generous in terms of her need rather than to feel inept in terms of his own. Bob was able to offer his wife a glimpse into his private world of grieving only after he acknowledged his right to grieve privately. Once his wife was reassured that he was experiencing grief, she could leave him alone. In each instance, these individuals were both mutually generous and at the same time true to their own temperaments. In each case, they were able to acknowledge and accept their different temperamental needs, and this acceptance of difference allowed them to remain comforting allies during the siege of cancer.

The Dynamics of Resolution and Some Suggestions

The *attitude* of the marriage partners comprises the starting point toward resolution. She can choose to see her husband as a mechanical, unfeeling and uninvolved deserter and remain caught in their relationship impasse. On the other hand, she can try to see him as an equally concerned partner dealing with the stress of cancer in his particular way. Should she choose the latter, she offers him an opportunity to trust her and to take the risk of behaving differently himself. He can choose to see her as a weak, incompetent and overreactive hysteric. On the other hand, he can try to see her in the truer light of a person dealing with the stress of cancer in her particular way. Should he choose the latter, he offers her the same opportunity to trust him and to risk a change in her behavior. Once they have chosen to regard each other with understanding and acceptance, they have taken that first step past the intolerable impasse. It is an immensely difficult step to take. She risks being bound by a schedule of his design, a blueprint without space for her to live emotionally.

He risks having to trust and depend on someone he often sees as being untrustworthy. And yet the potential rewards justify these risks.

To the extent that he is able, he can *listen* to her moods and keep repeating to himself, "I don't have to do anything, I don't have to solve anything, I don't even have to say anything to make her feel better." To the extent that he is able, he can give her brief reports about how he is feeling, not lengthy emotional discourses, but summary statements such as "I'm thinking about mom," or "I'm feeling blue," or even "I need to be alone now." He can try, at times, to assume some of the responsibility of initiating contact with his wife rather than waiting for her to woo him out of his quiet mood.

To the extent that she is able, she can respect his private world of feeling and thought. When he offers some insight into this inner world, she can let him know how helpful it is to her, and to the extent that she is able she can try to resist the temptation to dig for more. She might say to herself, "The more I demand and implore, the less he will reveal." She can try to make specific requests of him rather than using the "Why aren't you different?" type of criticism. And they can try not to play "balancing sheet," a destructive competition whose basic statement seems to be: "It's not fair, I do more than you do." Keeping a list of who does what for whom can be disastrous for the Hare-Tortoise couple since each contributes so differently in any given situation. Since it is their differences that furnish much of their strength, these criteria of "doing equally" can distort their genuine collaboration. Therefore, if they choose to be generous, they must throw away their checklists.

Jonathan[14] is a stiff and unexpressive man. He loves his wife, Samantha, with great devotion but cannot respond openly or be comfortable with her strong emotions. This becomes particularly problematic during the time in which her beloved father faces death. Not knowing how to help her, Jonathan tends to repeat the obvious: that all of us must eventually die, that papa is seventy-six and has had a long, rich life, that weeping cannot prevent his death. Samantha is experiencing deep grief, intense anger and a desperate need for her husband's warm support. She is also very sensitive to Jonathan's discomfort and disapproval of strong emotion and therefore faces a crucial choice. On the one hand, she can blame him for being uncomfortable and somewhat inept. She is very well versed at doing this. On the other hand, she can help him to "not just do something but stand there"; she can help him to understand and help her. For example, Samantha can explain how much comfort his holding her provides, how much she needs to be held and allowed to cry. She can validate their temperamental differences and express appreciation for his efforts to overcome personal inclinations and offer the support she asks of him. And she can expect him to be awkward and unpracticed with this new effort. There is a choice. Samantha can drift along (and face the consequences of that passive choice) or she can actively elect which area of feeling she wants most to experience at the moment. *Accusation* will lead to their typical confrontation, and she will have a familiar opportunity to express her "justified" anger. *Instruction* will help him to offer his "imperfect" support and emotional intimacy. In this case, she wanted and received an astonishing amount of loving comfort from a tentative but devoted Jonathan. There are many such choices for both husband and wife during the cancer crisis.

Another area of possible resolution has to do with assumptions. Since they do not share similar temperaments, they tend to make disastrous assumptions about each other. With the Hare-Tortoise couple, what is true for the goose is decidedly not true for the gander. During the siege of cancer, assumptions such as "She doesn't respect me," "She doesn't love me," "She thinks I'm a failure," "He doesn't find me attractive," "He doesn't think I'm trustworthy" or "He doesn't care" can serve as fuel for still more assumptions which produce bitter resentment and emotional stalemate. One of the most common areas of false assumption has to do with the emotions of hurt and anger. In the Hare-Tortoise relationship, she often feels hurt and covers this feeling with an angry attack; he often feels angry and covers his anger with a hurtful look. Predictable false assumptions accompany this masquerade. Since he is already well aware of her anger and she of his hurt pride, he would do better to let her know directly when he is angry and she more often to express her hurt feelings.

At times the couple with Hare-Tortoise tendencies are bound by their hope of changing one another. She refuses to abandon the hope of making him more emotional and open. He refuses to give up the idea that he can compel her to be more logical and calm. In fact, each clings to a cherished illusion. If they were to give up their hope of changing each other, they would have to admit that their ability to control each other's behavior is negligible. But it is clear that each partner in the Hare-Tortoise relationship can have much more of what he or she wants by not trying to change and control the other. This is so even when marital conflicts are cancer-related and there is a greater need for control.

These, then, are some of the problems that plague the Hare-Tortoise relationship during the siege of cancer. The couple are characterized primarily by their emotional differences, and these differences in turn provide their greatest opportunities and strengths. Let us now follow a couple with just such Hare-Tortoise tendencies through one of the most ravaging of all cancer experiences, the slow dying of a child.

The Story of One Family

I believe that Nancy Roach[15] and her husband Bob were able to give their daughter everything that parents are capable of offering. Their story illustrates a Hare-Tortoise couple who lived the cancer experience in an extraordinarily successful way, that is, they were able to develop their strengths and to satisfy their daughter Erin's needs. Nancy's account of how they managed the four and one-half years of Erin's illness is a beautiful testament to their love, understanding and courage. But it also illustrates their ability to weave the dramatically different aspects of their Hare-Tortoise temperaments into a profound marital union. Although it is one family's story, a great deal of the universal human experience is portrayed in Ms. Roach's narrative. It begins with the bewildering and tragic diagnosis of cancer when Erin was three years old.

When we heard "Erin has leukemia," it meant to us "Erin is going to die," and our grief began.

In looking back, this was by far the most difficult time for Bob and me. I spent the first two months crying—so consumed with self-pity I could not see to the needs of my sick child or devastated husband. Bob became engrossed in his projects. As he expressed it, "I just couldn't stand the thought of loving her and then losing her." Obviously we had a long way to grow.

They began by admitting their feelings to themselves and by using whatever means they could find to share them.

I have heard other mothers say they felt like they were riding an emotional yo-yo; securely held up at one moment only to be let way down the next. I experienced this feeling along with the prevailing sensation of sitting on top of a potentially eruptive volcano. At times the tension seemed unbearable, leading to what I have termed my "blonde wig syndrome." I would daydream about a quick and clever departure. Wearing a blonde wig I'd have a $25 paint job done on the car, equip it with old license plates and "split"—perhaps for Canada where I could get a job. This whole concept is totally incompatible with my nature but somehow the fantasy helped. I would arrive back to reality a little more rested from my mental vacation. . . .

There were many times during the four and a half years of Erin's illness that we were left without the time or energy to see or respond to each other's needs. Sometimes our misplaced anger was vented upon each other. When our tensions led to anger or arguing, we felt guilty because we hated to add another stress to Erin's already burdened life.

Communication was a problem. Initially, we found sharing our feelings extremely difficult. We were both protecting very sensitive areas within ourselves. We had to learn to communicate effectively if we were to pull together in our efforts to support Erin and each other. We began by writing notes because spoken words were sometimes too explosive. For example, if I felt Bob was spending time on a project to the exclusion of Erin and me at a time when we could have used some relief, such as an outing, my angry feelings would lead to a retaliation that would only turn him off. I found that when my anger had cooled and I wrote down my feelings, I usually ended up with a greater understanding of his feelings and my own. He would thoughtfully evaluate my written message and definite positive changes would occur.

We even found telephone conversations more effective because there were fewer distractions. In the later years, our ever-increasing ability to communicate (even if the words were sometimes angry) made our feelings easier to share. We had learned that we could put off our own needs for a better cause. We had become closer through our mutual sharing and concern over Erin's well being. Although we had friction, misunderstandings and frazzled nerves, there was a strong basis of mutual caring and the realization that we were two fragile human beings facing an enormous problem. In the end we knew that each of us had given all our love and had experienced together the deepest of human emotions. We learned to love unafraid. We had invested immense love and that love, we have learned, was not lost when Erin died. Rather, it became the better part of us.

In order to be able to "love unafraid," Nancy and Bob had to face the same intense experiences of denial, fear, anger and guilt that so many other couples must face. They began the weighty task of confronting these emotions firmly convinced that Erin's confidence and adjustment depended on their understanding and courage.

Understanding that Erin had leukemia was one thing; full realization and acceptance of the fact, we discovered, was quite another. Our denial of the total implications of the disease could be recognized in many ways. Initially Bob managed to keep himself very busy and distracted. I launched into my art work with greater determination than ever. On one occasion, Erin's doctor introduced us to another mother and her son saying, "You share a common problem." I found I did not want to see another child showing evidence of leukemia. This was too much reality for me. . . .

Bob and I were afraid—afraid of death and separation, afraid of not having made the best decisions about Erin's care and afraid of managing the seriousness of the disease on a practical level.

Before we could help Erin live with her illness and face her premature death, we had to confront these problems ourselves. It was terribly important that we shared with each other our feelings about death and how we would deal with Erin's dying. This was extremely hard because our feelings were so intense and we each felt the vulnerability of the other.

. . . Our feelings of anger were as intense as our fears. Why had this terrible thing happened to us? Why did our beautiful, bright little girl have to suffer and never grow up? We were angry at some powerful unknown, be it the forces of nature or an omnipotent God. We were angry at the doctors for their diagnosis. We were angry with friends and people who said insensitive things to us or who did not seem to understand what we were going through. We began to realize that our anger stemmed from our feelings of helplessness and frustration, and it started to diminish as we learned that there was really a great deal we could do. Even though we were powerless to change the fact that Erin had leukemia, we could support her, enjoy each day with her and make positive experiences out of potentially negative ones. This helped us toward a growing acceptance of life with all of its mysteries and challenges. It led to the realization that we are able to make choices and meet challenges.

. . . Almost as soon as Erin's illness was diagnosed, our self-recrimination began. What had we done to cause this disease? Was I careful enough during pregnancy? We knew radiation was a possible contributor; where had we taken Erin that she might have been exposed? I wondered about the toxic glue used in my advertising work or the silk screen ink used in my art work. Bob questioned the fumes from some wood preservatives used in a project. We analyzed everything—food, fumes, and TV. Fortunately most of these guilt feelings were relieved by knowledge and by meeting other parents whose leukemic children had been exposed to an entirely different environment. Initially, the self-blame led to a very unrealistic handling of Erin. We complied with her every demand to the extreme of responding to a midnight command for chocolate and cookies! This would have been appropriate for a child with only a few weeks to live, but obviously such a routine could not be sustained for a number of years without destroying Erin's spirit and our already taxed sense of balance. We began to realize we had to maintain a normal environment, but knowing her life would be short complicated our emotional response. If I resisted constantly playing games with her, I had a terrible sense of guilt and thought, "Some day I'll regret this." But realistically, she was sometimes impossible to play with. . . . I had to remember that a normal child would be encouraged to play fairly and independently, but it took me a long time to master my emotional response.

Since Bob and Nancy have very different temperaments their responses to the circumstances of Erin's illness were understandably different. Even the emotions of denial, fear, anger and guilt were experienced differently by each of them. But these differences were communicated, slowly accepted, eventually respected and finally utilized with great benefit. The Hare-Tortoise relationship pattern has the potential for endless tension and resentment. It also has the potential for the rich alliance that the Roaches were able to forge. Their willingness to face the fact of their different needs helped them to understand and respond to Erin's search for a child's understanding.

. . . Office visits revealed an important discovery—the more Erin knew and was able to express about her treatments, the better she managed. After returning home from a blood test, Erin worked through her fears by performing tests on Bob, me and her entire doll collection. She would stick our fingers and we would give an appropriate and realistic response, "Ouch!" She would then proceed with the test and we would ask questions. "Why are you taking a blood test?" "We are checking your blood to see if you are O.K.," she answered. "Why are you putting my blood on that little piece of glass?" "So we can put it under the microscope and look at it." Through this "instant replay," we were assured of her understanding, and she was reassured and less frightened of the unknown. . . .

Their recognition and respect for each other's differing temperaments made it more possible for them to support their daughter's unique experience of herself.

While she was recovering from a crisis during which she lost all of her hair, we played with hand puppets. Mine was an ugly alligator and Erin's, a beautiful rabbit. The alligator told the rabbit how terrible he felt about himself and Erin, through the rabbit, assured him that he needn't worry because he had lots of friends and people who loved and cared for him. She assured him that he had many special qualities shared by no one else.

Conversations such as these were vitally important. They gave permission to Erin's expression of doubt and distress and they provided her an opportunity to reassure herself with her mother's blessing.

Bob and Nancy were not intimidated by their own anger. They acknowledged it and found ways to express it constructively. Fortunately, they were able to pass this tolerance on to their daughter.

She had more than the usual frustrations and she had to find acceptable outlets for her anger. One of these was identifying with the little song from *Sesame Street*, "Now we're angry, very, very angry—REAL MAD!" Sometimes we lost both the patience and the objectivity to manage discipline problems effectively and at these times a family "blow up" would take place. . . .

. . . Erin fully understood her situation and needed to vent her hostilities. She had an excellent command of four-letter Anglo-Saxon words and used them appropriately during treatments. We had attempted to curb this in the past, but we came to realize that this was a good tool for her to use, and that we shouldn't deprive her of it—especially since her anger was so appropriate. One of the last things she asked of me was to teach her to write one of the more effective and potent of her favorite curse words. I agreed and together we wrote it.

The acceptance of their differing temperaments allowed them to bring the best of themselves to the complex demands of the cancer experience. They could augment rather than compete with one another. Bob's day-to-day help

> began when he arrived home from work. This was his special time with Erin. He gave her a bath and read the bedtime stories with far greater flourish than I could have mustered! This allowed me some time to be alone with my thoughts. If Erin had undergone medical treatment during the day and needed special rest, we all spent the evening together watching television, reading stories and even eating our dinner in her playroom.

Recognition and acceptance of their differences also made it possible for them to offer Erin a wider spectrum of positive parental attitudes. Nancy could share some of her daughter's deepest fears; Bob could let her frolic:

> Erin loved going to the playground, taking the wildest rides at the amusement park and swimming at her cousins'. Bob's sense of balance between freedom and caution was much better than mine. I tended to be over-anxious and purposely avoided some of these situations if he could take over. He allowed her to have fun but did not take his responsibility casually.

And Bob and Nancy's ability to accept help from each other made it easier for them to seek out and accept help from other parents in comparable circumstances.

> We found our greatest friend-support came from other parents going through, or having gone through, the same or similar illnesses with their children. We became involved in the founding of an organization called *The Candlelighter's Society,* the name being derived from the saying, "It is better to light one candle than to curse the darkness." . . . We knew we had a common problem and we shared our thoughts and feelings about the many different phases of the disease. We met parents who had already lost children and took strength from them. We found certain other people with whom we had a special rapport and could communicate our feelings on a deeper and more intimate level. We were amazed to find that our most frightening thoughts and fears were common to them as well. We shared our grief, pain, love and joy. I always felt more comfortable with "another mother" because I knew she really understood.

Bob and Nancy Roach were close allies when they faced Erin's approaching death. Their ability to recognize and accept each other's uniqueness made it possible for them to accept their fears, to speak of them, to cry together, to share philosophical visions (even with a child), and at the very end, to possess the strength and understanding to NOT interfere with Erin's private and personal adjustment to death, to let her guide them. Nancy's account captures the beauty of this family achievement.

Talking about death—even thinking about death—had always been difficult for me. Erin's illness brought me face-to-face with the most difficult death possible . . . that of my own child. The more I brought my thoughts and feelings to the conscious level, the easier the subject of death was to think and talk about. It was like flexing an unused muscle. As time went on, our conversations became more advanced. . . .

. . . Erin had met a little girl who came to the hospital to visit her brother who had leukemia. This little girl, Duney, was later to become Erin's best friend. Duney and her brother Michael played with Erin for many months. Then Michael became very sick and was no longer able to play. I began to prepare Erin for the inevitable. When we talked about how sick he was and about how he might not live much longer, her own inner strengths took over. She drew him pictures to cheer him and said things like, "At least I got to know him and play with him." The day he was admitted to the hospital in critical condition I told her he would soon die. The next morning we heard about his death. We cried together and talked about how much he had meant to us. I was glad we had shared everything and had not denied any of life's emotions. This complete sharing allowed us not only to feel the deep sorrow of a loss together, but also the intense joys, such as those brought about by a remission.

The days following Michael's death brought mutual consolation. If she cried, I would comfort her and when I expressed my grief, she would comfort me. This time Erin did draw an analogy between her own condition and Michael's. "Do Michael and I have the same disease?" "The name is the same, leukemia, but you have a different kind." (Michael had a very unusual type of leukemia that did not respond to treatment.) "He did not feel better with drugs and you do. You are able to feel well for long periods of time." At one point after a crisis during which she had many tests and transfusions and was thoroughly ravaged, she asked, "Does anyone ever get over this disease?" I answered, "You will always have to have treatment for it; so far there is no cure." "I know someone who got over it," she said. "Michael." I was surprised by this and said,

"But he died." "I know, but I would rather die than have any more back tests and stuff." At this time we had a very philosophic conversation about the quality of life. I asked her if she was not willing to go through some unpleasantness for some happy summer days of swimming and playing. She said, "I guess so." Time, in fact, did bring another remission and three more seasons of happiness.

. . . Conventional therapy was not working, a decision had to be made. Should we take the risk of administering more aggressive therapy (which could, in fact, shorten her life) or should we make her as comfortable as possible for the time she had left? While the doctors were making their decision, we felt it was necessary to share our concern with Erin and let her help us. The most difficult and yet beautiful communication was about to begin. She was drawing pictures on her bed tray and I sat next to her. "Erin," I began, "Do you know how worried we are about you?" "Yes," she answered. "Well," I continued, "the disease is not getting any better, and we have to talk about a few things." "Am I going to die?" "If you don't get into another remission you might. Here is the problem—maybe you will have another remission if the doctors use stronger drugs which could make you very sick." "You mean," she said, "it could kill me?" Fighting the tears I said "Yes . . . do you want to take the chance and all of the sticking for maybe some more happy days?" "I'd rather have the sticking and stuff than to die." "Thank you, Erin. This helps us to tell the doctors how you feel." At this point I had to excuse myself to blow my nose, but I returned to finish our talk. "Is there anything that frightens you that you want to talk about?" "Yes," she answered, "I'm scared I'll have to be here so long that you and daddy won't be able to stay any more." I quickly assured her that we would stay as long as she was there. Then I asked her if she was frightened about dying. She said that she wasn't scared of dying, but that she didn't want to leave us. I told her how much we didn't want her to go. She then talked about the friends she was going to see in heaven, and she wondered if God would let her sit on His lap. After this talk she was euphoric, as if she had been relieved of a tremendous burden. She seemed more equipped now to work toward her great task—dying.

And near the end:

. . . She no longer shared her feelings with us. When she said she was frightened we encouraged conversation, but she let us know in her own way that her feelings were now private and that she had a right to her privacy. We wanted so much to share her every thought and to be able to help her over to the other side . . . as we had done with every other phase of her life. But we knew this was something she had to do her own way. All we could do was to support this need by not interfering. She did not want any touching, kissing or loving, but she wanted us to be present. We stayed by her quietly. With her last ounce of energy she pushed my hand away as if to say, "I can do it myself." And early in the morning on the last day of April she died.

9

The Peacemaker Marriage Pattern

She is like me, part of my blood and we understand each
other . . . can't I make you see that a marriage can't go
on in any sort of peace unless two people are alike?
—Ashley Wilkes in *Gone With the Wind* by
MARGARET MITCHELL

Marriage of Gentle Similarities

We have reviewed and examined some of the essential aspects of the
Hare-Tortoise relationship. As with all complementary marriages, it
is characterized by temperamental *differences*. But what of the many
couples whose marriages are based more on *similarity* than difference from one another? I shall illustrate the patterns of these *symmetrical* relationships and compare them to those of the Hare-Tortoise
couple by using the familiar characters of Margaret Mitchell's *Gone
With the Wind*. [1]

Scarlett O'Hara and Ashley Wilkes never get married. But their
relationship admirably portrays the distinctive tendencies of the
Hare-Tortoise couple and suggests at least one of the reasons Ashley
chose his cousin Melanie instead of Scarlett. In this typical scene we
have an indication of what married life would have been like for
Ashley and Scarlett.

Scarlett, having heard that Ashley intends to marry his cousin
Melanie, decides to confess her intense, adolescent love. She waits

for him in the library, her heart racing. When he comes into the room she passionately declares herself. He is awkward and embarrassed, but tries to reason with her as she continues her unrestrained confession of love. He tries to be kind and reassuring but Scarlett insists that her love be acknowledged and taken seriously. Ashley lectures "Love isn't enough to make a successful marriage when two people are as different as we are." When Scarlett keeps questioning him about his feelings, about whether or not he loves Melanie, he insists ". . . that a marriage can't go on in any sort of peace unless the two people are alike." But Scarlett remains adamant. She reminds him of his flirtatious behavior, becomes angry and accuses him of being a cad.

Ashley is cold and quiet. He apologizes for any statements that might have led her to misunderstand his purely friendly intentions. He then adds: "How could I help caring for you who have all the passion for life that I have not? You who love and hate with a violence impossible to me." But she is not to be appeased by his distant admiration. She rages at him "Why don't you say it, you coward! You're afraid to marry me! You'd rather live with that stupid little fool who can't open her mouth except to say yes or no. . . ." Ashley pleads with her to be fair but she springs to her feet screaming "I'll hate you till I die, I can't think of anything bad enough to call you" and slaps him with all her strength. He becomes stiff, cold and withdrawn, says nothing, leaves the room and, with rage spent, Scarlett is left feeling desolate. Rhett Butler is also in the library, unobserved, and he has been listening to their conversation. When she is startled by his presence and accuses him of not being a gentleman, he roguishly teases her: "An apt observation. And you Miss, are no lady." He will later insist that they are exactly alike.

Here then we have our cast of characters. Scarlett and Ashley confront one another in the way we have come to expect two people sharing a Hare-Tortoise relationship to behave: she passionately accusing him, he silently suffering her accusations, nobly waiting for her to realize that he is really a good man. Although Scarlett is in love with him and Ashley is in awe of her intensely emotional nature, although they are attracted in precisely the way that opposites attract one another, they do not marry. He sternly believes that a peaceful marriage is achieved only when the two partners are alike. This refined, considerate, reasonable and dispassionate man therefore marries his refined, considerate, reasonable and dispassionate cousin Melanie. And eventually the passionate, mistrustful, competitive and emotional Scarlett marries the equally fiery, competitive, mistrustful and confronting blockade runner, Rhett Butler. Each is identified with his or her spouse, each tends to borrow from and fuse with the other, each tends to see their personal qualities reflected with varying degrees of acceptance in one another's behavior.

Ashley and Melanie live their peaceful marriage without ever exchanging an angry word; Rhett and Scarlett live their stormy one, rarely sharing an unguarded moment. And each couple manages to avoid a large area of life's experience. These popular literary marriages may serve admirably as an introduction to the next relationship patterns we will consider. Ashley and Melanie are the Peacemakers; Scarlett and Rhett are the Gladiators. Each type of relationship has its strengths and weaknesses and each can lead to predictable problems, especially during the stress of cancer treatment.

Peacemaker Characteristics and Cancer-Related Stress

Couples who share similarities with Ashley and Melanie are characterized by their consideration and thoughtfulness, by their friendliness and generosity and by the peacefulness of their marriages.[2] They are nice people who rarely argue, rarely state strong preferences, rarely say no to any request, and tend to define an "ideal marriage" as one without friction. They are good people and, during the cancer crisis, they are probably the most vulnerable to depression.

Ralph and Joyce[3] had been married for nearly fifteen years. Their youngest daughter Beth had leukemia and she was in her third remission when Beth's physician referred them for counseling. They were desperate. They could not imagine how they were going to

continue taking care of her. Each felt enormously guilty and emotionally depleted, and each felt responsible for the crisis. A great
deal of anxiety came from their belief that the other was also helplessly ineffective in dealing with the demanding circumstances. They
had elevated Beth's physician to a godlike stature and were asking
him to make almost all of their decisions. Ralph saw himself as
hopelessly inept by comparison. His wife shared this view of him and
secretly resented her husband's sad declarations of incompetency.
Each became more and more depressed and refused to believe the
other's reassuring words; each was equally convinced that the other
spouse neither respected nor loved him. They came for help not
knowing how to go on. An understanding of the Peacemaker relationship pattern will help us to understand how Ralph and Joyce fell
into their paralyzing depression and what they might have done to
prevent it.

Peacemakers are usually raised in families that detest difference.
They marry others who equate difference with dangerous disruption
and thereby create new families that detest difference as well. The
lives of Peacemakers are relatively free of conflict but suffused with
a chronic fear of *losing control,* of being *rejected* and of exposing their
anger. These same three areas of vulnerability, as we have seen, are
intensified by the stress of cancer treatment, and they affect each
relationship pattern differently.

Peacemaker Emotional Strategies and Loss of Control

A great many of the Peacemakers' decisions are intended to avoid
confrontation with anything that might prove to be unpleasant. By
rarely having strong opinions or dislikes, each hopes to escape criticism and disapproval; by being as inoffensive as possible, each hopes
to be overlooked by danger. However, during the siege of cancer,
the danger can no longer be avoided and their lives threaten to rage
out of control. Peacemakers attempt to deal with this "dangerous"
loss of control by the selective use of guilt, by assuming emotional

responsibility for everything that occurs and by an assumption of moral superiority. Each strategy can backfire and lead to depression.

The Exploitation of Guilt and Generosity. Peacemakers are well practiced in the use of guilt. They have a lifelong tendency to use it as justification for reward: "If I've sacrificed enough I'll be worthy of love and acceptance." They use guilt to disown responsibility for unwanted feelings and thoughts: "I'm sorry to be in such a dreadful mood; I really didn't mean what I said." And they also use it to induce obligation: "I'm feeling so bad (so weak, so sad, so helpless)," implying that it would be criminal to refuse whatever it is they are asking for. The use of guilt is among the most effective strategies that can be employed in the attempt to maintain a sense of control. It is used to some extent by almost everyone. But there is so much guilt associated with the image of cancer that an overwhelming sense of unworthiness and a corresponding inability to accept help may accompany the Peacemaker's habitual attempt to maintain control by exploiting this emotion. Unable to accept help from each other, Peacemakers often search for absolution through giving. They assume responsibility for everything, cannot do enough for others and often become overburdened, resentful and exhausted. Instead of absolution, they then experience even greater guilt. This is especially true with the demanding circumstances of cancer treatment. Each claims responsibility for all the problems and insists that his or her spouse is the kindest, most considerate person alive. Together they sink into a state of depressed helplessness and berate themselves for their failures.

The Hidden Illusion of Power. The statement "It's all my fault" suggests more than guilt. It reveals an illusion many of us share but few are aware of. If we believe that we are to blame for the problems we encounter, we also imagine that we are capable of resolving them. We cannot hold ourselves accountable for their continuation unless we assume the power to reverse their effect. Whether we realize it or not, this illusion of transcendent power usually lies hidden below our confessions of failure and leads directly to guilt and depression. Peacemakers are especially gifted at suffering the consequences of attempting to be responsible for everything. On one level, they rarely say no to any request, they feel they should be able to solve the problems of others and they immediately respond to the unhappiness of a friend or family member with an offer of some kind. If they are unable to resolve the difficulty, they protect their illusion of power by assuming that their failure rests in some particular fault of their character. Their guilt expresses this compelling notion. To care about people and not be able to help them gives rise to sadness and great sympathy. But *guilt* issues from the pretense to godlike powers and the failure to attain them. There is much more here than the desire to be benevolent. The secret assumption of omnipotence promises complete control over the unknown, and the heavy burden of guilt and depression that is reported by so many peacemakers derives from the misguided belief that the power is still available, if only they can correct some failing in themselves.

The need to experience a sense of control is extreme when patient and family face the problems associated with cancer treatment. It is not surprising that this hidden illusion of transcendent power asserts itself to compensate for the bewildering experience of helplessness. It is common for cancer patients and their families to harbor fantasies of magically curing the illness, of exorcising surgical defects and of generously bestowing lost happiness and security. But the assumption of total responsibility must inevitably lead to the experience of total failure. And this is particularly true for Peacemakers since both husband and wife share these tendencies toward illusions of omnipotence and corresponding guilt.

The Misuse of Moral Superiority. Under these stressful conditions, many Peacemakers assume a tone of moral superiority. A rarely voiced, self-righteous contempt emerges when pain and confusion are the Peacemaker's only rewards for having assumed too much responsibility. If the frustration and outrage are consciously felt, the Peacemaker patient or spouse can finally justify the long-restrained desire to make demands. Now that he or she can claim to be the victim of a great injustice, the long-suppressed outrage erupts. The intimidated spouse is barraged with complaints and demands. Unfortunately, the Peacemaker who erupts into a self-righteous martyr can only continue to justify his or her behavior by continuing to suffer. And so a dreadful cycle is established: suffering, "justifiable" demands, remorse, guilt, and further self-imposed suffering sufficient to justify another wave of miserable outrage. But under this defensive moral superiority lie envy and the wish to unburden oneself. It would be a great deal easier for Peacemakers to do so if they were not also afraid of rejection and their images of abandonment.

Peacemaker Emotional Strategies and Fear of Abandonment

Individuals who marry and evolve Peacemaker relationships have always feared criticism, disapproval and potential rejection. They have therefore adopted recognizable strategies to avoid these anticipated "catastrophes." Being extremely sweet, generous and nice, rarely stating strong opinions, showing a great deal of concern for others and assuming enormous amounts of responsibility are some of the ways they hope to inspire obligation and to ward off potential rejection. Charm and consistent friendliness are the Peacemakers' stock in trade. The kind and generous offers of Peacemakers are usually sincere. But we are interested here in the way it comes about that those engaged in Peacemaker relationships are *exclusively* sweet, nice, generous and considerate. I am suggesting that intense fears of disapproval and rejection are largely responsible for these patterns.

Peacemakers have always attempted to banish the normal resentments, criticisms and negative feelings that are a natural part of being alive. But, during the cancer crisis, they must deal with an inner raging protest of great intensity. The sweet generosity of the Peacemakers could not withstand the growing anger and the accompanying threat of rejection which they feel were it not for a particular distortion of reality most Peacemakers unknowingly employ during times of stress. They fall prey to an exaggerated sense of their partners' fragility.

The Perception of Fragility. The conclusions drawn from the sense of another's fragility might be stated as follows: "If I'm not careful with him, he'll fall apart." Once this assumption has been made the Peacemaker is spared the necessity of being direct and honest about negative feelings. After all, Peacemakers reason: "If my wife is so delicate and unsure of herself (or if my husband is so easily hurt), I most certainly cannot be direct and honest. I really have no choice—I must be generous and sweet." There are safety and purpose in these mutually held disparaging images. In the context of such fragility, the anger and raging resentment, so much a part of the cancer crisis, are seen as especially dangerous and therefore must be suppressed. However, the suppression of so much anger and resentment (out of misguided protectiveness and fear of rejection) inevitably leads to depression.

If the stress remains minimal or if it is intense but of short duration, the sweet, considerate, loving support easily given by one Peacemaker to another is enormously helpful. But the stress may be unbearably intensified when only "acceptable" feelings are expressed over a long period of tension. Peacemakers then tend to deal with the escalating tension by believing themselves to be more fragile than they really are. They must then begin to experience themselves as trapped victims.

Ralph and Joyce became depressed in precisely this manner. Their ordered and pleasant life was thrown into disarray by their daughter's diagnosis. When both their chronically lurking fears of rejection and their long-suppressed marital resentments were magnified by the cancer crisis, each assumed an almost superhuman amount of responsibility. They both became depressed and progressively more guilty as Beth remained seriously ill, and their relationship began to deteriorate under the strain of their sweet generosity and silent suffering. Rather than share the rage and the irrational, the vivid resentments and personal grief, each blamed himself for having failed and desperately tried to save the marriage by exaggerating his sense of personal fragility and soliciting the other's sympathy. In fact, their great vulnerability to the threat of rejection derived, in part, from a marital history of partial intimacy.

Untested Intimacy. Since Ralph and Joyce had only shown each other their sweet and generous faces and had rarely, if ever, participated in an angry exchange, they came to know a gentle but extremely tenuous kind of intimacy. Having carefully screened disruptive qualities out of their lives, their intimate relationship remained untested. Since they had never confronted one another, they could not know what might happen if they ever did. They were therefore in a difficult position from which to confront and share their inner turmoil. This innocence of conflict can be even more of a problem when a spouse, rather than a child or parent, is being treated for cancer.

Peacemakers attempt to feel worthy of love and respect by being good, generous, kind and considerate. That these attempts are usually vigorous and one-dimensional is a reflection of underlying feelings of unworthiness. When cancer is diagnosed it is most often experienced with great shame, as if those hidden and unwanted feelings beneath the sweet generosity were "finally exposed." The image of abandonment then looms up and is experienced as a deserved punishment. In this respect, Peacemakers are no different from most people. The "shadow" experience is widespread, frequently reported and usually followed by the fear of rejection. But the Peacemakers share a temperament and a role. They have established a symmetrical relationship and they are therefore vulnerable to this "shadow" experience in a correspondingly unique way. Given the gentleness, concern and generosity characteristic of Peacemakers, we would assume that they would also share an ideal emotional environment in which to reassure and comfort one another. But, unfortunately, it is precisely these familiar and generous qualities that often lead them toward estrangement.

When cancer patients are in Peacemaker relationships and experience rage, shame and repugnance for themselves, they tend automatically to assume that their spouses feel exactly the same way about them. Since they have always agreed about important things, have always shared each other's needs, values, and goals, and have always colluded with each other in not expressing what might be disruptive or hurtful, this assumption is quite consistent with the way they have always perceived and dealt with one another. How easy it then is to discount and dismiss the reassurance offered; how easy to believe that the "truth" must be so terrible it dare not be revealed. And, since negative feelings and thoughts have always been banished, the cancer patient becomes more and more convinced that these intensely judgmental feelings must also be experienced by the spouse. The chronic fear of abandonment, now made acute by the stress of cancer treatment, makes it even more difficult to state real fears, ask direct questions, or believe reassuring replies, and under these circumstances mistrust grows stronger. We can see how the long-standing Peacemaker choice to avoid expressions of resentment, disappointment and disapproval has led to an atmosphere of growing insecurity. The impact of what has *never* been said contributes to a wall of vigilant disbelief. It is not surprising that alarming fantasies multiply and create a certainty of abandonment out of these undiscussed assumptions of condemnation and disapproval. The sweet generosity of the Peacemaker couple often leads, in just this manner, to intense anxiety during the cancer crisis.

Banished Anger. Peacemakers are rarely aware of a conscious choice to legislate anger out of their lives. But this choice has been made. They are also often unaware that they live in accordance with strict rules regulating the expression of hostility, but these rules exist. Although unstated, they often include the following injunctions: "Do not show anger. If that proves impossible, disguise it. Avoid confrontation. If unavoidable, act condescending." During the cancer crisis, Peacemakers strive for peace at any price. They try to behave in a manner that they think others will admire. But, in the process, they often achieve a shallow and unconvincing peace; tension, resentment and misunderstanding often lie beneath the sweet words and generous offers they exchange. This shallow, peaceful existence is an attempt to eliminate the fear that a "terrible truth" lies hidden in the shadows below. To be angry is to risk a return of anger. Peacemakers simply will not tolerate the idea of such emotional disruption, for it might lead to the devastating confrontation of which they are so terrified. Children of couples who share these Peacemaker tendencies often report that, during a time of stress, they feel like they are living with two "time bombs." They remain tense and afraid but, given the family rules, must always remain sweet and considerate and must never comment on their great discomfort or vivid perceptions.

Peacemakers believe they haven't the right to feel resentful or angry even when they are experiencing these emotions. When we consider all of the sources of resentment and anger associated with the cancer crisis, we can vividly imagine how painful it must be for the Peacemaker to be caught in so much conflict. Every other relationship pattern described has at least one person capable of expressing strong feelings. But to the Peacemakers, such a response always seems too irrational and too inappropriate. As a result, they soon begin to feel trapped, taken advantage of and burdened with their ambitious efforts to make others feel comfortable. An inner protest grows more intense but their Peacemaker rules forbid expression of it.

If the anger and resentment associated with cancer treatment are suppressed, great tension results. The suppressed anger will turn inward and cause feelings of depression and helplessness. Given these Peacemaker patterns of interaction and the predictable problems that derive from them, how can couples who share these tendencies prevent depression and helpless despair from adding yet another burden to the cancer crisis?

Resolving the Peacemaker Marital Impasse

When the Peacemaker roles are themselves contributing to the stress of cancer treatment, they obviously need to be modified. Two major tasks arise whenever such a modification is attempted; Peacemakers must become acquainted with feelings and acts they consider inappropriate and they must give up many of the safe advantages of their Peacemaker roles. Such risks always seem monumental; resentment, criticism, disapproval and disappointment might emerge. The same frightening image of rejection that has persuaded them to control their negative feelings for so many years is still as threatening. The unknown still seems as forbidding as ever. But when the Peacemaker roles fail during the cancer crisis and the weight of helpless depression begins to descend, many couples are willing to experience the anxiety of taking risks and are willing to work toward a stronger, if stormier, alliance.

The Process of Change. The first step in the process is the acknowledgment of what is being experienced, regardless of whether it seems unreasonable, irrational, inappropriate or terrible. The next step is to develop a curiosity about the presence of these unwanted feelings, to trust that one is not a monster for having them, and then to explore their context, discover the rhyme and reason for their unwelcome appearance. Once they are acknowledged and accepted, it is necessary to give the feelings some form of expression. It is certainly possible to do so without blaming or condemning a spouse. When an open and nonblaming atmosphere exists, feelings such as disappointment, resentment, sadness, irrational rage and doubt can be fully described and each Peacemaker can hear, possibly for the first time, the whole story of his relationship. A new trust can be built in this manner, a trust that fosters deeper personal recognition since it bases itself on authentic acceptance of oneself and of a loved one.

Lucy had been married to Gil for nearly twenty years when she had a mastectomy and underwent radiation therapy.[4] I talked with him during Lucy's treatment and he was obviously extremely worried about her: "She has always been frail. Why do the good people seem to suffer more than the others? She's never had it easy, she's always had to struggle. You know, she has worked hard and given us all so much. . . . At times it seemed like the kids and I pulled her down, like a heavy weight."

If we listen carefully below his worry and distress, we can hear some of the themes that suggest the Peacemaker pattern: the assumption of fragility and injustice, the implied responsibility for her suffering and the accompanying guilt. But Gil and Lucy did not allow themselves to remain frozen in Peacemaker roles. They realized through the stress of Lucy's treatment that, although they were very happy with each other, they were also dissatisfied with certain aspects of their marriage. They decided to try to change what might be causing this disturbing, if minimal, estrangement. They could not have known when they entered family therapy that several months later they would be daring to confront one another in so vigorous a manner. In one tense hour, they said many of the forbidden and unthinkable phrases that each had always denied or pushed aside. Gil was the first to acknowledge and express his "inappropriate feelings."

GIL: . . . This makes no sense but I really resent you for getting sick. I know it's not your fault, Lucy, but at times I actually hate you for being sick and putting the burden on me. . . .

LUCY: . . . but that's so unfair (begins to cry). I didn't want this to happen. I can't help it, you know that.

GIL: I know how hard this has been for you but some things just aren't right. I go around grumbling to myself all the time. [*Grumble out loud, so Lucy can hear you.*] . . . She whines and complains all the time. She doesn't do much and I don't mean housework. She could start getting up more, start seeing people more, going out, doing things like she used to do. [*How does all this affect you?*] I feel lonely, like with an invalid, and I resent all the extra things I have to do. I think you take advantage of the fact that I never refuse you anything. It doesn't seem fair to me either.

LUCY: I am trying. I push myself a lot. Gil, please don't be mad. I'm really trying. It's just not fair to do this to me now. [*What did you hear Gil saying?*] That I'm whiny and lazy and self-indulgent, that he doesn't like me this way. [*See if that's what he means.*] Isn't that what you're telling me?

GIL: In a way. I'm so tired of tiptoeing around the house, tired of seeing you feeling sorry for yourself. I guess I don't like you when you're acting this way. [*Lucy, what's happening in you, right now?*]

LUCY: I've always done everything for him, I've tried to please him. I have been a good wife, you know, a very good wife, and now when I'm sick and recovering from cancer, now when I really need him, he's acting like this. [*Like what?*] Like he's deserting me. [*And how does that make you feel?*] Sad. It makes me sad and want to cry. [*Anything else?*] Well, it doesn't seem fair. [*And when Gil is being unfair, I feel . . . can you go on?*] . . . He's not so perfect either. I've always overlooked lots of things. [*Tell him a few of them.*] Well, for one thing, I'm always tiptoeing around too. If I say anything the least bit critical, you go around the house moping just like Billy used to do when he was four. You never notice all that I do for you, but every little thing you do you want a special citation for . . . (tense pause). This is scary. [*What are you afraid of?*] I don't know what Gil is thinking. [*Ask him.*] I really shot my mouth off, didn't I? . . . Are you very upset?

GIL: No, but it's not easy to listen to these things. . . . Since you've been sick, I've been doing everything. [*Right now, do you want Lucy to be sweet or honest?*] I want to know, I want her to be honest. [*Do you believe him?*]

LUCY: No . . . [*Tell him why not.*] Because you never want me to say anything that will hurt your feelings. You know that.

GIL: Right now I don't want you to be a poor suffering martyr. [*Maybe you could tell her some of your resentments?*] There's one main one: I get so tired of all your little problems. You go on and on about them for hours. You never just ask me to do something. I'm always having to play Mr. Wizard to try to figure out what it is you're hinting at that I'm supposed to do.

LUCY: Mr. Wizard! If for once you'd just stand up for yourself . . .

I had obviously succeeded in provoking them. The banished voices of their marriage had begun to speak out and to be heard. They were acknowledging their feelings and describing them. And, even though it is nearly impossible to do so without at first blaming each other, they were beginning to describe their fuller experience of married life. Before this moment, they had treated each other as fragile playmates, as carefully indeed, as they had indicated they wished to be treated themselves. They had both tiptoed around the other's "fragile ego." But their exaggerated fragility, their sweetness and their guilty assumption of endless responsibility had masked many down-to-earth human resentments. Lucy's illness became almost irrelevant; their love as well as their resentment had existed before her treatment and it continued in similar form after it. But, although they were well versed in the art of peacemaking, they also became quite capable of stepping outside these habitual patterns of polite avoidance. Sweetness had covered a reservoir of small but real resentment. These grievances could be discussed by them at great length and with a growing ability to accept the feelings and not blame each other for their presence.

Lucy and Gil went on to discover that not only was their un-remarkable resentment covered by a blanket of false cheerfulness, but that under their resentment there existed a great many additional feelings that had also been unknowingly banished as what they felt to be inappropriate. He talked about his fears; his financial worries because of the unexpected costs of treatment and hospitalization; of how he feared for her life, afraid that she would just give up and die, that he would be unable to keep her spirits up, that she would stop loving him. He talked about how much he valued their years to-gether. And Lucy was able to describe her fear that he would leave her, that her sadness and disfigurement were repugnant to him and were driving him away. The closeness and trust that grew out of these intimate conversations were completely new to them. They came to believe that their past dedication to "peace at any price" had served as an obstacle to this new and valued experience of intimacy. Gil and Lucy, by their openness and courage, had not only prevented an escalation of the problems inherent in their Peacemaker relation-ship pattern, but they had used the opportunity of the crisis to achieve a richer and more supportive marriage.

The Essential Conflict. Peacemakers typically exploit their depen-dency as an effective means of emotionally binding their marriage partner. In the process, however, they sacrifice or diminish their personal authority and competence. If they have practiced these tactics in the past, they are ready for use during the cancer crisis. An understandable conflict then emerges. If Peacemakers turn to their personal strengths and face the tasks of cancer treatment, they reveal these strengths to their spouses and disrupt a successful system based on niceness, fragility and dependency. Gil exposed his independent abilities and found himself alone with overwhelming responsibili-ties. A great emotional leverage was lost in his Peacemaker relation-ship pattern when "too much" personal authority and competence were revealed. Lucy risked the advantages of being "poor Lucy" when she began to confront him. But, if the Peacemaker turns away from these personal strengths out of fear of losing control or being abandoned, he or she is left truly helpless and can all too easily become depressed. A helpless victim like Lucy is often a Peacemaker who has *chosen* to sacrifice all semblance of personal authority and competence in a desperate attempt to feel safe and protected. Having made this choice, the poor Peacemaker is compelled to become more childlike, more helpless and more dependent. Choosing to regard one another as responsible adults, capable of hearing a full range of emotions, is the essential first step toward resolution of the Peacemaker impasse.

10

The Gladiator Marriage Pattern

And of what value is the grain of sand at the heart of a pearl.

—RICHARD ADAMS, *Shardik*

The Fight for Love and Respect

Just as Ashley and Melanie were our literary prototypes of the Peacemakers, Scarlett and Rhett may serve admirably as models for the Gladiators. As a couple, they form a dramatic contrast to Ashley and Melanie in lifestyle. It would never have occurred to them to think of each other as vulnerable or fragile. Rhett would never have attempted to protect Scarlett from the harsh or turbulent realities of her life. And Scarlett, regardless of pain or loss incurred, would not customarily have been kind or generous to him. Neither of them was ever compelled to be protectively polite to the other. They criticized, disapproved, bullied, blamed, ridiculed and threatened one another for the many years of their marriage. Although Rhett was immediately, and forever thereafter, strongly drawn to Scarlett's passion and strength, he provoked and taunted her from the moment they met. And, although Scarlett was consistently drawn to Rhett's powerful presence, she rarely stopped insulting him. Whereas Ashley and Melanie saw in one another that which they aspired to be, Rhett and Scarlett saw in one another that which they both *admired* AND *disliked* in themselves.

Although they were completely at home with the turbulence of their continuous conflict, they could not tolerate even the beginnings of those close, open and trusting moments for which each secretly yearned. Like all couples with Gladiator tendencies, these tender emotions filled them with anxiety and alarm.

Rhett and Scarlett were armed fighters. They longed to be at peace together but each insisted that the other disarm first. And, even when one dared to begin to do so, the other could not believe the authenticity of the gesture. The inevitable response to such gentle offers of tenderness, compassion or generosity was an even more guarded and mistrustful challenge. Consequently, they lived a series of near misses. His kindness and generosity could occur when she was overtly rejecting, but if Scarlett responded with warm affection, she could expect to be greeted by his sarcasm. And yet, after every long siege of silence or separation, one of them would return with a flicker of renewed hope. Over and over again they would beat upon the locked door that barred the way to the love and comfort they so ardently and ambivalently fought each other for.

Social scientists, like the rest of us, observe such sad battles with dismay, especially during the stress accompanying serious illness. "Some spouses, both men and women, are overtly hostile . . . not only do they give no help, but post-operatively they may add to the patient's difficulties. . . . They give the appearance of great interest and solicitude for the patient in the early phases, but their subsequent behavior reveals the true nature of their feelings. They give minimal or no help post-operatively and are frankly hostile and rejective."[1] But why have such couples stayed together for so long? Does this overtly hostile behavior really show "the nature of their true feelings"? In most instances, I do not believe that this is so. Their Gladiator relationship prevents them from behaving in a supportive and loving manner, but knowledge of the Gladiator tendencies can help all of us to understand the reality that often exists beneath the battle cry. And, once understood, it is possible for peace negotiations to succeed in creating allies during the siege of cancer.

Gladiator Characteristics and Cancer-Related Stress

Gladiator relationship patterns are characterized by their long-term combat. Every issue of married life is another potential area for conflict: politics, how to raise children, sex, the defects in each other's character, the qualities of each other's friends, where to take a vacation—it hardly matters. The goal is to feel superior, to be right, to triumph. Therefore Gladiators must always be on guard and they must never admit doubt. They must also vigilantly hide their true longings, for these can be used against them in the next bitter encounter. They long to hear their spouses capitulate, to admit finally that they were wrong, that they had been fools and provocateurs and that they are now prepared to love and adore and make up for all their misguided attacks. Each has the same hope, the same wounds, similar doubts and fears, the same tender need for love and respect, and each covers these feelings with endless hostile accusations. Hostility and tension become the matrix of their lives and, like anything familiar, even this marital warfare becomes ritualized and safe. But, given the paltry rewards for all the effort, why do Gladiators stay together? There are several reasons.

In the first place each is dependent on a strong rival. Should they divorce and remarry or should one of them have an affair with someone who possesses the very qualities they accuse one another of lacking; if they begin to live with someone who is quiet, gentle, appreciative and generous, they invariably become bored and experience their lives as dull, empty and without meaning. They hunger for human contact but only seem to be able to experience it temporarily in the excitement of heated competition. A widow expressed this vividly: "We used to fight all the time. Nobody could understand why we stayed together. I'll tell you the truth, I left three times and don't even know why I went back. But now he's dead and I don't have anywhere to go. I don't even have anywhere I want to go . . . who else would put up with me?"[2]

The fierceness of their battle is a reflection of their need for one another. They can become so identified that they lose all awareness of the boundary that separates them and might afford them a sense of independent selfhood. Despite their armor and their style of fighting, the loss of this personal boundary makes them almost as vulnerable to stress as the Peacemakers. Instead of forbidding criticism, anger and disapproval, they manage to exclude tenderness, trust and generosity. Each becomes so identified with his or her hated rival that they merge as one in battle. A threat to one of them is a threat to them both, and when threatened they fight each other with all their might.

The Paradox of Gladiator Confrontation

Despite their belligerent denials, most couples who possess these Gladiator tendencies are afraid of being abandoned. Most know the fear that goes with the statement "Who else would put up with me?" And, since they have exchanged so much cruel abuse, they are especially prone to feel retroactive guilt during the cancer crisis. The *patient* often feels defeated and anticipates rejection as a "deserved punishment." The *spouse* feels the guilty remorse of the victorious survivor, the inexplicable discomfort of imagining that he or she has driven a spouse into a serious illness and therefore must anticipate a comparably painful punishment. Fear of abandonment, as we have seen, is a common aspect of the cancer experience. But Gladiators have their distinctive response to this fear. They watch for any signs of rejection and then retaliate with all their aggressive strength. Once again, they use their practiced ability to fight as a means of warding off anxiety. However, during the cancer crisis this strategy creates a tragic paradox as they unknowingly attempt to drive others away out of fear that they might themselves be rejected. A cancer patient says: "I let my kids have it. They came one time and didn't have two words to say. You tell me what kind of kids don't even talk to their father at a time like this."[3] The wife of a cancer patient says: "Sometimes I actually feel like he went and did this to me. We fought a lot but, you know, there were lots of things I couldn't give him. Not only children, but being a more interesting person. But then he says something nasty and I get furious."[4] Both of these people feel hurt but cover this feeling with a barricade of anger.

It is very difficult for Gladiators to experience the pain, sadness and need for love that lie beneath the surface of their belligerent accusations. They find the feelings of gentleness and tenderness intolerable because they awaken a sense of vulnerability. Perhaps their greatest fear is that of falling into a deep depression. A cancer patient says: "I've been a fighter my whole life but then this happened to me and I began to feel—what the hell's the use? I started giving up."[5] This man had always assumed that there were only fighting and "giving up." For him, not to be a fighter was not to exist. This is a frequent experience for Gladiators, who enter into combat in order to keep ahead of a nagging sense of meaninglessness. If they become seriously ill and can no longer actively employ their distinctive, combative style, they begin to experience a depression that has always stalked their footsteps. Many Gladiators provoke their raging battles in a heroic effort to distract this lurking despair.

The husband of an exhausted cancer patient confesses: "We used to keep each other going. I can't seem to do it by myself. I feel like I'm slipping down. Even the things that I do well, like my teaching, seem to be getting heavy. Since Mary is so weak, I'm sinking down with her."[6] Pain and sadness are often experienced by both marriage partners when their battle is interrupted. But the expenditure of energy needed to maintain the distracting conflict, especially during the cancer crisis, can be exhausting and may also lead directly to depression. And so the Gladiators face a terrible dilemma: they are each prone to depression if they stop fighting and the fears of the cancer experience make them yearn for comfort, love and recognition. Yet, precisely because of this yearning and its accompanying sense of vulnerability, they begin to fight like mad. They drive friends, family members, health professionals and each other to exasperation with their antagonistic outbursts. They fight with everyone until they are exhausted. And then they become depressed, having never confronted their fears of intimacy and vulnerability.

The Price of Victory

Winning the war has always promised great fulfillment to Gladiators. They can fight for years in an effort to come out on top. But, if one of them "breaks" during the stress of cancer treatment and the other is finally the winner, the victory is almost always experienced as loneliness, remorse and depression. Here is another paradox of the Gladiators' struggle; even when a victory is achieved (and it doesn't matter who has won) both become depressed and experience a lonely isolation.

It is a rare Gladiator who does not feel doubt and uncertainty. Fighting for an ultimate victory and trying to dominate the other is a reflection of pervasive self-doubt. The unknowns of cancer treatment deprive all patients and their families of a needed sense of being in control. But Gladiators, who expend enormous amounts of energy striving to prove themselves superior, who are constantly toiling to regain a sense of control through intimidation, are more vulnerable and more shaken than others. It is harder for them to accept uncertainty and there is no way for them to avoid it. They find themselves bewildered and in acute conflict, fighting fiercely to prove themselves superior to cancer or to a spouse with cancer. The *patient* vainly tries to control a disease which he or she experiences as an inner weakness, an unworthy trait now blatantly evident in the form of cancer. Since total victory has been established as the only criterion for success, the uncertainties of cancer treatment often lead Gladiators to a feeling of defeat and total failure. The *spouse* in turn usually reports a sense of extreme frustration. Gladiators attempt to gain control by means of armored attack. But, since the cancer is in another person, a spouse cannot "get at it" and begins to feel uncertain and inept. As a consequence, he or she attacks the patient with renewed vigor and frustrated rage. As the fighting escalates, the underlying yearning for support, recognition and comfort gets lost in the heat of battle.

Gladiators are not plagued with the emotional burden of unexpressed anger. Each knows well the wrath of the other. But a great deal of their fighting does not represent anger. With them, stated grievance has become well-rehearsed ritual. Their alienation remains on the surface while their mock battles distort far deeper needs. They are lonely warriors who suffer the emotional burdens of disowned tenderness and unexpressed love. But there are emotional bridges available for them if they choose to use them. These are not easy alternatives. They require admitting to areas of fear and anxiety, enduring the stress of closeness and taking the first tentative steps toward trusting the habitual rival.

The Turning Point

Tom and Evelyn[7] had been married for fifteen years when she underwent a hysterectomy for uterine cancer. He was a busy doctor who had, for many years, openly declared his marriage a disappointing failure. In his eyes, Evelyn was a conventional housewife, without imagination or a flair for living. He saw her as a "complacent" sexual partner, as someone who did not care to improve their "mediocre existence." Evelyn had been a nurse when she fell in love with Tom, whom she saw as a "handsome and ambitious" young intern. But her infatuation quickly faded; she became furious with her new husband and bitterly disappointed with her marriage. In her eyes, Tom was inept, blaming and deceitful. She viewed his grievance as "nothing but adolescent nonsense" and believed that this naïveté about life revealed Tom's "pathetic immaturity." Their family sculpture illustrated these experiences of one another. Evelyn had him sitting in a variety of passive postures while she busily took care of the kids. In each pose he would say, "Get me the paper" or "Where are my glasses?" or "Keep the noise down," while she fumed with anger. In his sculpture, Tom placed her at some distance before him and had her raise a stiff arm each time he approached. Evelyn's rejecting movement was accompanied by the statement "Don't bother me." They both had a gift for characterizing the other's inadequacies and "reprehensible" characteristics; both felt that they had never gotten what they needed from the marriage. And yet neither had ever made a serious move to separate.

After Evelyn's cancer treatment, the familiar competition over who would give in to the demands of the other became more intense. Each felt greater deprivation, and this led to frustration and bitter outrage. Evelyn vacillated between a childlike withdrawal and angry criticism of Tom. He, in turn, taunted her for being depressed and threatened to leave when she became abusive. The first steps toward changing their Gladiator responses to one another occurred during a tense and revealing conversation. The exchange followed many hours in which each tried to prove that the other was the responsible villain. It was the first time that they had been willing to step beyond their ritualized complaints.

TOM: I don't know what to do any more. She's depressed and somehow wants me to come up with some miracle answer to her problems. But every suggestion I make gets a disgusted look or a nasty putdown. And, of course, if anything goes wrong it's my fault.

EVELYN: Do you think spending all day preparing a lavish meal for our friends is such a brilliant idea? For God's sake, Tom, I can't even keep up with what I have to do. You complain we don't do anything, but if I don't make all the arrangements, pursue every last detail, then nothing happens. You want so damn much and you don't do a damn thing.

TOM: I work sixty hours a week and come home to a hassle. I can't even catch my breath for two seconds in my own house. [*Tom, imagine walking up to your front door after a day's work, what are you feeling and thinking? Say it out loud so Evelyn can hear.*] What problem is it going to be this time? What's the latest thing she's going to complain about? What thing didn't I do right this time? How much has she suffered today? [*And how am I feeling about all these things?*] Shitty. I almost wish I were going anywhere else but home. All I want is some peace and quiet. If only once she'd greet me with a smile, fix me a drink and keep the kids off my back for an hour or so, so I could relax . . . but when I open the door, I know that look on her face and I think, here we go again.[*So if I were in your shoes, I'd open the door already disappointed, resentful, and prepared for the next battle.*] Sure. Why should today be different than any other day? [*Evelyn, when you know Tom is due home, what are you feeling and thinking?*]

EVELYN: Help! That's just what I'm feeling. I need some help. If someone could just take care of the kids for a while, just give me a little break before dinner, but I know what he'll be saying. "I'm so tired, Evy, do this, do that." I haven't had two minutes to myself all day long and now I've got another one who wants me to take care of him. . . . [*So if I'm Evelyn, I'm already resentful and saying No as he comes through the door.*] Sure. We've been through it a million times. [*And if you are particularly put out, how do you let him know that you think he is a bastard?*] I don't know. I tell him. [*But how do you go about it? How can you really get to him?*] . . . He is always forgetting things, so I throw them at him. I let him know how miserable I've been and how it's mostly his fault. (A little laugh.) He comes in feeling like a big shot. He's been out helping everyone in the world and I start telling him how much he doesn't do, for me and for the kids, how much he isn't even capable of doing. I'm cold and turned off to him. [*A pretty potent arsenal. Are they familiar to you, Tom?*]

TOM: You bet. And she's left out a whole bunch of them. [*Like what?*] . . . Like being interested in me, in my work, in what's really happening in my life. Like keeping herself attractive. [*We've heard from Evy and now you've started. Can you say more about how you make her feel lousy about herself?*] I only complain when I'm frustrated and angry. [*And, as you've said, you believe it's Evelyn's fault. So how do you get back at her? Be really honest and tell her what your weapons are.*] I let her know what a drag it is living with her. What a conventional, boring housewife she is. I tell her that she's lost her looks and her charm. How many beautiful women are hot for me and how much more they have to offer me. I let her know that I'm tempted. . . . I also put her down sexually [*How?*] By not being at all satisfied even when she tries not to be inhibited. [*Even when you are satisfied?*] Sometimes. [*I now want you both to do something that isn't going to be easy. Here are some of your weapons, right here in front of us. Imagine, for a moment, not using any of them. Look at one another and imagine not having them to protect yourself with, and then tell each other what that would be like for you.*] (Long pause.)

EVELYN: You mean if I didn't put Tom down? . . . I'd be scared. I'd feel naked. [*What would you be most afraid of?*] That he'd be right. And that would mean that I'm nothing. Just a dumpy, complaining nuisance. [*And if you begin to feel like a dumpy, complaining nuisance, what might happen?*] I'd have to admit that he really doesn't care and has good reason not to. I'd get really depressed and he'd probably leave me. . . . I just thought of something. I never thought of it this way before but I think that as long as he's not feeling sure of himself he's afraid to go. So I keep putting him down. [*Finish the sentence and say it to Tom —If I let you begin to feel good about yourself . . .*] . . . There's no reason for you to stay with me. (Tears.) . . . [*But why would you be upset if he* left?] . . . Because I love him. [*Can you say that to Tom?*] No. It's been too long. [*How do you think he'll respond?*] I don't know. . . . [*What do you see when you look at him right now?*] He's uncomfortable. [*Are you curious at all about what he's feeling?*] I'm afraid. [*Take a chance and ask.*] (She looks up at him.) Tom—I don't know what to say. [*Tell Evy what her tears are touching in you.*]

TOM: I start to feel trapped. . . . I don't know. Mostly I want to get away. [*Are you feeling sad?*] Sort of. [*Try and tell Evy about the sadness and doubt in your life.*] It's hard to describe. I'm alone so much of the time, always surrounded by people and yet all alone. So much of the time nothing seems real. I feel like I'm passing through my life and not touching it. It's there for a moment and then it's all unreal again. It all sounds so stupid. I've got a successful career, a wife, healthy children, but I don't know, something isn't there. . . . [*See if Evy understands what you're trying to say.*] Do you?

EVELYN: I'm not sure. I see you're unhappy and I feel it must be my fault.

TOM: I blame you a lot. I imagine that another woman, an exciting affair, will make me feel more alive, a little more real. But I suspect it probably wouldn't. It's something that's missing in me. . . .

Under the familiar accusations of their endless battle, Evelyn and Tom felt sadness, doubt, loneliness and guilt. As soon as they stopped blaming each other for their fears and disappointments, for their sadness and loneliness, they began blaming themselves. It is therefore not surprising that within a few days they reclaimed their weapons and resumed their familiar warfare. But the first break in their well-practiced pattern had been made. They had defined the defensive use of their fighting tactics, admitted their vulnerability, and for a moment they had experienced the frightening possibilities of unguarded intimacy. But much work was still required of each— Evelyn had to confront post-operative fear of rejection; she had to begin to ask herself why she had never developed her dormant abilities. Tom had to face his "aloneness" and begin to resolve his lifelong conflict about commitment. They gradually minimized their blaming and slowly began to trust each other in a way that enabled them to share the deeper struggles in each of their lives with growing empathy. In the past, every event had been an opportunity for them to attack each other. But each momentary victory for Tom or

Evelyn was another defeat for them as a couple. By giving up many of their tactical weapons they were able to lower an emotional drawbridge and allow the other, for the first time, to enter their heavily guarded inner fortress. Once inside, they began to know the tender and unprotected spaces that each had hidden from the other.

Gladiators face a critical choice during the cancer crisis. They can retain their armor and weaponry or try, like Tom and Evelyn, to create a bridge toward trust and closeness. The pattern of endless confrontation in Gladiator relationships is probably the most difficult to alter. For many people, the exposure of sadness, doubt, grief, helplessness and loneliness is just too dangerous. They prefer the control and safety of carefully guarded emotional isolation, and they handle the cancer experience much more effectively this way. Other Gladiators choose to take advantage of the opportunities inherent in the stress of cancer treatment to reach beyond the limitations of their well-rehearsed roles and well-practiced competitiveness. It is a frightening prospect for Gladiators to face each other without their armor and many panic during disarmament talks; to trust is to be extremely vulnerable, and no rewards can be guaranteed. There are only opportunities, choices, risks and predictable consequences if no change is attempted. The risks and opportunities are worth consideration by any couple who possess strong Gladiator tendencies.

11

The Parent-Child Marriage Pattern

> Therefore shall a man leave his father and his mother, and shall cleave unto his wife.
>
> —Genesis 1:24

Training in Responsibility, Training in Trust

The Parent-Child marriage pattern characterizes many marriages in our culture. When reciprocal and experienced in moderation, it can offer great comfort to both husband and wife. However, predictable problems can be anticipated during the cancer crisis.

Whether by emulation of a distinctive parent, or by filling in the vacuum left by an absent or negligent one, some of us acquired an early education in how to assume responsibility for the care of others. In doing so we learned to be self-assured in positions of responsibility. But, since we had little practice in trusting or relying on others, we have remained uneasy when forced to depend on them. On the other hand, there are those of us who, having been able to bask in the glow of a mother's nurturing love (or a father's protective adoration), were understandably reluctant to give up our "land of milk and honey." In doing so, we learned to trust and rely on others, but neglected to develop our independent sense of personal authority and competence. When such a gratified son or daughter marries someone who has been well trained in the art of being a good and responsible parent, the resulting marriage has many characteristics of a Parent-Child relationship. There are marriages in which a great deal of mother-son interaction occurs and those in which the father-daughter dynamics are pervasive. Each pattern has its advantages and disadvantages and each has areas of strength and vulnerability that emerge during the cancer crisis.

Parent-Child Characteristics and Cancer-Related Stress

Parent-Child marriages are characterized by well-defined roles. They are often extremely stable and successful, for the roles that each willingly and comfortably enacts satisfy the majority of their respective needs. Husband and wife are able to anticipate and support each other. They experience a familiar identity and each knows what is expected. Both therefore feel a minimum of uncertainty about themselves and each other. But problems arise when their well-defined roles prove insufficient to some new circumstance or crisis. Then, the underdeveloped and neglected aspects of each partner's personality are exposed and each may become confused and vulnerable.

When change is mandated by circumstance, those in parent roles, although struggling to maintain their sense of independent competence and control must let themselves be taken care of by others. It is not easy for them to do. And those in the more childlike roles, who might be desperately struggling to maintain their sense of protected safety, must ask themselves to experience an unfamiliar aloneness, assume alarmingly new responsibilities and be willing to make independent and fallible decisions. These roles, which offer an unusual degree of stability and comfort during less stressful times, can become debilitating obstacles to family continuity when they resist modification during the stress of cancer treatment. Let us examine how these relationship patterns function under ideal circumstances and how they can break down during unfavorable ones, how each spouse might experience the strain of such relationship deterioration and what preventive opportunities each has at his or her disposal during the cancer crisis.

Mother-Son Relationship Tendencies. Mother-Son relationship tendencies can provide an enormous amount of strength for a family as long as mom remains strong enough to stay in charge of their lives. Milton and Sarah[1] were in their late sixties when he was told that he had lung cancer. He had always been extremely dependent on his wife; she was the one to make important family decisions, to reassure him in business pursuits and to resolve the daily problems of their lives. She was willing to do so and was certainly capable of playing this role. A strong, competent woman, she went with him to the doctors, arranged for his hospitalization, buoyed up his spirits and even became quite knowledgeable about cancer treatment. He returned home, was tenderly and maternally nursed by his wife, recovered without incident and their lives continued without significant disruption. Sarah's evident strengths dovetailed perfectly with Milton's needs and with the temporary demands of the cancer crisis. Milton and Sarah had weathered stressful events in the past and they handled the strain of his cancer treatment with characteristic harmony. But what happens when "mother" cannot fulfill the demands of her role? What happens when circumstances require each to perform unfamiliar tasks in relation to one another? Kathy and Doug, a younger couple with whom I worked, had a marriage pattern remarkably similar to that of Milton and Sarah. Unfortunately they did not fare as well.

Kathy was forty-six years old when she was told that the small lump in her breast was cancer.[2] She had a radical mastectomy and also underwent preventive radiation therapy. A persistent infection prolonged her convalescence, but she has been free of cancer for the past eight years. Kathy's most vivid and disturbing memory of "that time" is not the surgery, radiation therapy, wound infection or even her physical disfigurement. It is her memory of the "unbearable feeling of helplessness" she recalls during her recuperation. The Mother-Son marriage pattern can help us understand how this woman's "helplessness" could have been experienced as the worst part of cancer treatment.

As we have seen, the image of cancer evokes forbidding fantasies; it arouses issues of control, fears of abandonment and ambivalent responses to evoked anger. Cancer treatment further intensifies these fears and anxieties. Kathy, who had identified herself so vigorously with her mother image, and Doug, who had remained in many respects a lovable but dependent child-husband, were both vulnerable to these sources of anxiety.

Kathy rarely felt uncertain prior to her diagnosis of cancer. She had clear and fixed expectations of herself, her husband and her children. She was good at what she did and experienced her strength and capability. She could be extremely assertive and could confront anyone who had effect on the quality of her family's life. She was also adept at fighting away her own doubts and conflicts. But, since she had successfully avoided circumstances that made her feel unsure or mildly out of control, she was completely unprepared for the cancer experience. "I'd never felt so panicked. I didn't know what to do and this was strange to me. You see, usually I have a good idea of what I should be doing. . . . I knew I had to go to the hospital, but . . . I don't know how to explain it other than to say I didn't know what I was doing. I was so scared and I didn't even know what I was scared of. . . . I really didn't think I would die but I didn't know what was going to happen." Kathy was experiencing the other side of her highly developed competence and control; the part she had refused to acknowledge. She was now in an extremely unfamiliar position both with regard to the external realities of hospitalization and the inner realities of uncertainty, dependence and vulnerability. Her panic was in direct proportion to her long-standing unwillingness to be taken care of by others and to her chronic aversion to the experience of uncertainty. Her panic issued from the emergence of a disowned part of herself.

Kathy became depressed during her recuperation. "That time seems unreal to me. I can remember thinking I was nothing but a draining blob. . . . Doug looked lost and I would sit around thinking, 'I'm useless, good for nothing.' I tried to get active but would feel exhausted, then I'd feel even worse. I just couldn't do anything and it was horrible. It's hard to believe how depressed I felt, but I remember it well." A "Supermom" needs to be needed; she needs

to experience herself as indispensable to her family. She is dependent on their dependence on her. In addition to having lost an
important sense of control over her life because of her cancer treatment, fatigue took away her ability to care for her family and thereby
threatened her primary source of self-worth. Although Kathy knew
that Doug and the kids "really" cared for her, her depression was
augmented by a catastrophic fear that, because she could not take
care of them, she was worthless and would soon be unwanted.
Whereas some women esteem themselves for their sexual attractiveness or vivacious personalities, a "Supermom" takes great pride and
pleasure in her formidable capacity to care for others. The threatened loss of Kathy's ability to perform these duties constituted an
intolerable anguish; her fundamental justification for feeling worthy
of love and respect seemed absent. It is not surprising that she
remembers her recuperation with such abhorrence.

   Doug's experience of his wife's cancer treatment was just as stressful but very different. He had chosen a wife who was eager to take
care of him and he had remained at a job that was routine and
undemanding. Throughout adult life he had managed to avoid many
parental and marital responsibilities by being cooperative, supportive and understanding; by being a "good man at heart" whose
feelings could be easily hurt. When he learned that Kathy had cancer, he turned to her, as always, for help and guidance. But as
treatment and recuperation dragged on, Kathy became less and less
available and he was faced with independent responsibilities for the
first time in his life. "I remember everyone asking me questions. I
didn't know what to do. It seemed as if I had lost my bearings. Our
world was falling apart and Kathy got really depressed. I didn't want
to bother her. . . . I didn't know how to help her. [*What were you
afraid of?*] I was sure I'd do everything wrong. All I could think
about was how much longer it would be until she was all right again
and I wouldn't have all the pressure on me. I was ashamed to be so
selfish but that's what I kept thinking."

   Doug also had paid a price for the benefits of his role in their
Parent-Child marriage. He had remained in a childlike, dependent
position, and without Kathy's guidance he felt sure he would do

everything wrong. Doug, like anyone in a child role, expected himself to fail when confronted with a major responsibility. The cancer crisis threatened his protected sanctuary, and it is therefore not surprising that he found himself in a world "falling apart," deprived of confidence and independent judgment and lost without Kathy's maternal guidance. Doug's anxiety drove him into greater and greater dependency, and when Kathy could not comfort, reassure and take care of his needs, he lost his bearings. An important force contributing to his anxiety was the rage attending his enormous disappointment. Each of us who accepts the role of child in a Parent-Child marriage elects to exchange emerging independence and the development of personal competence for the "guarantee" of always being taken care of. When this implicit promise of protection is betrayed, raging disappointment and retaliatory protest make it difficult to assume new and necessary tasks during the cancer crisis.

Kathy and Doug had been comforted and reassured for many years by the well-defined and mutually satisfying roles each had developed. However, unlike Sarah and Milton, they could not be sustained by these roles during the cancer crisis. Since they had depended exclusively on their familiar expectations of one another, they became confused and depressed in circumstances that required a modification of their relationship. Kathy and Doug were unable to comfort one another in large part because they refused to accept the new requirements and responsibilities of their altered circumstances. Kathy could not bear her incapacitation; Doug refused to accept his new marital and parental duties. Their Mother-Son relationship tendency had always contained the potential for such a breakdown, and Kathy's cancer treatment provided the specific precipitating stress. The "Achilles heel" of their marital relationship lay hidden in the grossly disproportionate arrangement by which they shared responsibilities.

Since many of the same Mother-Son themes apply to Father-Daughter marriage patterns in inverted form, we will consider these tendencies before examining the available means of resolving or preventing the potential stress inherent in all Parent-Child relationship patterns.

Father-Daughter Relationship Tendencies. A husband who assumes the role of "Benevolent Big Daddy" to his wife has many of his most pressing needs satisfied. He is respected, praised and depended upon; he rarely experiences uncertainty or personal vulnerability. But his sense of confidence and control depend upon his wife's admiration; it is her adoring glances and needful requests that help maintain his sense of himself as exclusively wise, kind, strong and lovable. His father role is not only predicated on her supportive responses, but on his continuing ability to stay "on top of everything." Herein, of course, lies his greatest potential vulnerability.

During the cancer crisis, a patient who has always played this role will fight against being dependent on anyone and struggle to regain his sense of control and self-confidence. But in the many instances when he simply cannot do this, the heavy burdens of being "Big Daddy" begin to exhaust him; his fatigue and undeniable feeling of vulnerability then throw him into greater panic and fear. The wife of a cancer patient says: "I can't get him to rest. I've never seen Pete so worked up and stubborn. The doctor orders him, I beg him, but he can't sit still or let anyone do anything for him." Her husband replies in private: "My whole world is slipping through my fingers, you can't imagine what that's like. I know if I don't push myself I'll have lost it forever. [*What do you imagine would happen if you took care of yourself more?*] I am taking care of myself and I know what will happen if I stop pushing. I'll be a tired old man, I'll be finished and I'm not ready for that yet. [*How about Ann?*] Don't let Ann kid you. She can't stand to see me this way. She says, 'I'll take care of things,' but she can't stand it. [*And what if she is sincere? What if she really wants to take care of you for a change?*] Don't you believe it. I know her and I know what she needs. She's always needed me to take care of her."[3]

But why is Pete so unwilling to allow even the possibility that a genuine change might be in progress? Like most husbands in a Father-Daughter marriage pattern, he needs his wife's childlike helplessness to bolster his self-esteem. He therefore attempts to keep their roles intact. The "whole world" that he reports slipping through his fingers is the familiar and supportive world of his acknowledged dominance. Pete insists on taking care of himself in the area most crucial to him; he insists upon the restoration of his role as "Big Daddy."

The husband in a Father role rarely gets angry. He is more often a gentle lecturer. The rage following cancer treatment is therefore directed at himself and his growing sense of weakness. Pete's frantic behavior was an effort to stave off his lurking self-doubt, a task that became more difficult as he grew more and more angry at himself.

The potential for such extensive loss of self-esteem and resulting depression is inherent in every Parent-Child relationship. We strike a hopeful bargain whenever we use another person to build up our self-esteem, but we also guarantee ourselves a status of perpetual vulnerability. We receive support, admiration and reassurance and come to see ourselves as more than we seem in our own eyes. But we must continue to rely on others to judge our worthiness. Having given away the authority to assess, criticize and esteem ourselves, we find it impossible to avoid becoming hopelessly dependent upon the one to whom we have delegated that authority. A crisis occurs when the external source of self-esteem becomes unavailable or when another's assessment is adjusted downward. Not only is the extra measure of self-esteem lost, but very often so too is the entire sense of one's self-worth. The potential for such depression is an important part of the Parent-Child marriage pattern. In this instance, a husband has used his wife's girlish admiration to inflate his sense of manly self-worth, and when he can no longer fulfill the role that inspired her adoring responses and she begins to scold him for being unreasonable, he is in jeopardy of experiencing the complete collapse of his self-esteem.

A woman who is "adopted" by her husband usually experiences her marriage as a sanctuary that protects her from the stressful demands of an indifferent world. Her husband's presence offers a reassuring buffer, a place to be small and adorable, a retreat in which it is possible to love and to trust. A Father-Daughter pattern is not restricted to timid, childlike girls. There are many capable women who choose such a marriage as an emotional complement to their careers. Their qualities of strength, competence and decisiveness may be quite conspicuous in the world at large, but in the role of wife they undergo a strange transformation to helplessness, ineptitude and vulnerability. Women who venture into the world of self-fulfillment and responsibility may share many relationship characteristics with those who never leave the home; it is possible for both to take alarm and seek refuge under their husbands' protective, parental wing.

Childlike wives are much more in control of things than they or their husbands like to admit. Their adorable, exaggerated vulnerability is extremely effective and they usually get what they want from their protective husbands. In actuality, he is not as wise or strong and she is not as helpless as they both pretend. But, since the roles of the Father-Daughter marriage pattern are extremely satisfying for both husband and wife, marriages that contain these tendencies are unusually stable, and neither spouse challenges the other's role. When a child-wife is afraid to be alone or is disproportionately unsure of herself, the husband reassures her and she covets his reassurance. But, as we have seen in the Mother-Son pattern, there are specific dangers during the cancer crisis for those who commit themselves to this type of relationship, and these problems emerge when their Parent-Child system is seriously disrupted.

Summary. Whereas all of us feel despair at the loss or potential loss of a loved one, those involved in relationships with strong Parent-Child tendencies are burdened with an extra measure of dependence. We are speaking here of degree. All of us desire and try to attain family relationships of trust and devotion, of safety and comfort, but to the extent that we place the source of our self-esteem or our ability to survive in the hands of others, to just that extent are we dependent upon them for our sense of self-worth and survival. Parent-Child marriage patterns contain an extreme degree of this kind of dependence. Those who assume parent roles struggle with issues of self-esteem and control, those in child roles more often with issues of survival and fear of failure. The areas of vulnerability are correspondingly magnified when either the wife or the husband is threatened with the loss of a marriage partner. One experiences a threat to his self-esteem, the other to his ability to survive independently. The threat is as emotionally disproportionate as was their original overdependence upon one another. Resolution of this problem can only be achieved when the couple are willing to share responsibility in a new and demanding way and when they begin to reestablish personal ownership of the sources of their individual integrity.

Resolving the Parent-Child Marital Impasse

Ben and Carol[4] had been married for nearly fifteen years when he underwent extensive surgery of the palate because of a malignant tumor. He was ten years older than Carol and they shared many Father-Daughter relationship tendencies. Ben was a kind and competent man, looked up to by his business associates and by his wife. He was tender and protective of Carol and tended to assume most of the responsibilities for the family. She adored him and said she had never felt safe or happy until they had been married. Carol usually got what she wanted by being coy and playfully seductive. She was extremely frightened after Ben's surgery and made numerous frantic calls to the hospital. But within weeks Ben had recovered from surgery, mastered a prosthetic device, was able to reassure her, resumed his Father role, and despite the stress they settled down to their normal routine and pattern. Or did they?

Carol could not push aside her experience of extreme vulnerability during Ben's cancer treatment. The stressful shock had exposed so much dependency and alarm that she was no longer able to believe in the protected sanctuary provided by her fatherlike husband. When the panic subsided, the seeds of worry implanted during the cancer crisis began to grow. Carol became increasingly aware of her extreme dependence upon Ben and began to initiate changes in their marriage. At first the efforts were modest and Ben encouraged them. With time and growing confidence, however, she began to pursue more independent ventures: new friendships, personal interests, a job, success, growing responsibilities. She began to emerge as a genuinely self-assured and independent woman, and at that point Ben began trying to restrict her activities. Carol's insistence on her right to emotional independence caused conflict and anxiety in both of them. Their marriage became strained and they sought counseling.

Carol had withdrawn much of her affection from Ben. She was guarded, distant and stubborn; her greatest fear was that she might slip back into the old relationship. "Three years ago I was much too insecure to get a job, let alone get one and not turn to Ben for help. I was sure I'd fail. I'm still scared that I won't make it on my own, but I can't bear the thought of being the way I was." Carol's new belief in herself was tentative, her sense of independence still emerging and unclear. She was therefore extremely threatened by Ben's affectionate pressure on her to be, once again, a lovable protected child; she became increasingly stubborn and withdrawn. When Ben realized that he could no longer control Carol's efforts toward the establishment of greater personal authority, he became more and more anxious and could only perceive her rejection. When he realized that he could no longer intimidate her, he tried to fulfill all of her needs by making grandiose offers of time, gifts and help. Ben was willing to accompany her anywhere for any reason. She steadfastly refused his offers. In fact, she resented his "helpful" calls and appearances. He could not desist and said: "I just can't bear to think of her getting into the awful problems I can prevent." I asked him what three adjectives best described his present experience of the marriage. He replied: "Inadequate, threatened, and panicked." Ben was sure that she was "leaving" him because he had somehow failed her and that she would soon fall in love with a younger, more capable man.

Over a period of months each came to understand their marital struggle as an expression of the Parent-Child tendencies of their relationship. Ben began to appreciate the enormous burden of Carol's undertaking and Carol could appreciate his anxiety and distress. They became allies in bringing about a change in their marriage. Several months later, Ben got a call from Carol, who was on a business trip in the Midwest, wondering if he cared to join her for a few days' vacation. He caught the next plane. They had a wonderful time in this "neutral territory," made love "like in the old days" and felt closer than they had for many years. Ben had given her the space to pursue her career and independent interests. He had been able to manage his loss and anxiety. Carol had begun to believe the sincerity of his effort and was therefore able to be close and loving again. But she was guarded when they returned. The remodeling of a long-standing marriage pattern takes time; her reserve following the vacation reflects the incompleteness of this process. But the essential perspective had been established. Ben finally understood what was being accomplished, they were both able to tolerate the loss of their familiar safe roles and the desired change in their relationship was achieved.

There is an epilogue to the story of Ben and Carol. Two years after their family therapy, Ben underwent a second cancer operation. His convalescence was longer and more complex but the stress each experienced was significantly reduced. The frantic, childlike wife (who had called the hospital so many times each day and in such panic six years before) no longer existed. The fatherlike husband (who had to quickly reassure her and immediately resume all of his prodigious responsibilities) was also greatly altered. In their places were two people devoted to one another and able to share the tasks of cancer treatment. Carol's mature, tender love was a gift Ben had never imagined possible. Her support and the comfort they could now offer one another is a testament to the courage with which they faced the stress of change.

Parent-Child marriage patterns can be changed when they no longer provide comfort. Change is certainly possible but it is difficult, painful and often discouraging. I have not portrayed the many underlying conflicts that can occur. But we must all anticipate these unique obstacles whenever we attempt to bring about a new form of family support.

Summary of the Sphere of Family Influence

Complementary marriage patterns are characterized by differences in the marriage partners. Hare-Tortoise and Parent-Child patterns illustrate such complementary relationship tendencies. *Symmetrical* patterns reflect similarities of temperament in the marriage partners. Peacemaker and Gladiator relationships demonstrate two contrasting possibilities. Complementary relationship tendencies have their strengths and weaknesses during times of stress. So do symmetrical ones. In fact, all patterns of relationships (those described in the previous chapter and the many that have not been mentioned, those that illustrate marriage relationships and many others that illustrate larger family units) are capable of being supportive, generous, productive and meaningful. All relationships (and most are a blending of these patterns) are also capable of escalating the stress of cancer treatment.

The relationship tendencies presented in this section may serve to illustrate general marital patterns. They also suggest ways in which individual family members may approach identifiable problems. However, they can only provide a blueprint for change when change seems in the best interest of those who suffer. The responsibility for change remains with each of us. The ultimate value of these patterns can be no greater than the new goals and behaviors which they encourage. But, once inaugurated, the process of change can be dramatic and enormously gratifying. It can change a hopeless and embittered family environment into one of closeness, warmth and exciting growth.

PART FOUR

The Search for Meaning

In *Part One* of this book, I endeavored to portray the many facets
of the cancer experience: fears of the unknown; struggles with
anxiety, abandonment and the shadow side; the hidden bond
between depression and anger; and the importance of mourning.
Part Two took us beyond these experiences and introduced the
many areas of potential personal influence that can be exerted
over them. In *Part Three,* I presented some distinctive
relationship patterns that can have great effect on family life
during the cancer crisis and described several means of resolution
for the predictable emotional stress that can occur. The cancer
crisis is often experienced as a burden to be endured. It is even
more often experienced as punishment for sinful transgression. If
we were to conclude with these understandings and strategies of
adaptation, we would have failed to acknowledge the most
significant life-affirming force in existence. There is another
dimension that is characteristic of those who triumph over tragic
circumstances: *the ability to grow beyond the crisis of cancer by finding
a personal meaning within it.* The search for such meaning and the
many forms in which it can be experienced will be the subject of
this last section.

12

Beyond Crime and Punishment

A single moment can retroactively flood an entire life
with meaning.
  —VICTOR E. FRANKL, *The Doctor and the Soul*

Crusaders and Victims

To look beneath the surface of despair is to find a suffering without
significance. There can be no better definition of victim than "one
who suffers without purpose." The soldier in combat faces fear and
hardship. He knows his life to be in grave danger and often experiences the pain of physical and emotional impairment. But when the
fear, hardship, pain and possible death are seen as a heroic sacrifice
for some deeply held belief or are experienced in the context of the
comradeship of shared suffering, the deprivation can become profoundly meaningful. It is experienced in a manner that transcends
personal comfort and individual life. Pain and discomfort become
much more than mere pain and discomfort. Actions are undertaken
at great peril to life, not only through obedience to authority, but
in accordance with personal belief and purpose. Although such convictions cannot be maintained at all times, the awareness of larger
purpose gives sustenance to the overall effort. But there are circumstances in which no such meaning exists.

Consider another soldier in combat, one who sees the war as

senseless, immoral and without guiding principles, one who perceives the enemy with needs and aspirations similar to his own. This soldier will experience the discomforts, pain, dangers and risks in a completely different manner. Although he suffers the same conditions, he will despair of his meaningless suffering. Two soldiers in similar circumstances: one proud crusader, one depressed victim. These two totally different experiences derive from the presence or absence of meaning, not from the external conditions of war.

Despair regularly attends stressful conditions when no purpose can be found for suffering. The dynamics of personal meaning illustrated by these two soldiers are similar to those experienced in the crisis of cancer treatment. But here the individual tasks and the evolution of a deeply felt, subjective significance are much more difficult; no national cause is promoted, no grand purpose is immediately apparent and the sufferer is often isolated. Today it is more difficult than ever before to find meaning in suffering.

The Reflecting Mirror of Meaning

The personal search for meaning has a distinctly contemporary quality. A great deal of purpose was experienced in the act of suffering by those of our grandparents' generation. Most believed that if they faced adversity with courage, faith and acceptance, a higher power would acknowledge such effort, render judgment and provide eternal rewards. But, in our rational and scientific age, there is diminishing social validation for the belief in a life after death. One of the casualties of our scientific dedication has been the loss of meaning traditionally associated with suffering. Without such belief, pain is only pain, loss is only a feeling of terrible loss and death promises no pathway to a richer existence. There are many people today who hold genuine religious belief, but there are also many who feel spiritually orphaned and demand a highly personal sense of significance from life itself.

The question of meaning becomes intensely relevant when we are faced with the possibility of our own death or that of a loved one.

A near, possible death assumes the form of a reflecting mirror, forcing us to behold the unexamined values by which we have been living. Such confrontation, although disruptive and frightening, allows us to shift our attention from the superficial to the profound and to touch the core of our existence. The intense light which radiates from our own potential death causes some of us to shut our eyes while others use it to view life with greater clarity. The cancer crisis has been reported as just such an illuminating experience by countless patients and their families. They begin to reflect upon values, goals and commitments. They become involved in a process in which this deeper perspective reveals certain values as provisional and others as truly sustaining. The cancer crisis is rarely a time for radical change. But it is an excellent opportunity for serious contemplation. Individual values emerge in a new light. When the crisis has passed, one person elects to live her life with grace, discipline and dignity. Another discovers the Carl Sandburg verse "I've been a good man and done what was expected;/Now I'll be an old bum, loved and unrespected," and follows this inclination. Each of us has a task, a personal meaning at the core of our life. Or, as Emily Dickinson expressed it:

> Each life converges to some center—
> Expressed—or still—
> Exists in every human nature
> A goal.

Stressful circumstances can foster the search for this center of significance by requiring us to open ourselves to the fullest range of life's possibilities.

The Subjective Phenomena of Meaning

When a family is assaulted by the diagnosis and treatment of cancer, they become, at first, enmeshed in the confusion, irrationality and chaos that so often accompany these circumstances. Philosophical speculation can be bitter and cynical; no meaning can be found in the tragic events; external design and purpose are not apparent. The eventual evolution of meaning must be a completely subjective process; indeed, the experience of meaning in this respect clearly resembles the subjective phenomenon of pain. The only general conclusion drawn from a review of 687 scientific studies designed to investigate the character of physical pain was that it could not be scientifically characterized; pain could only be defined "as every man defines it introspectively for himself."[1] In other words, pain is what it is experienced to be. These studies force upon us the astonishing awareness that pain may be extremely intense despite the fact that there is no scientific proof it exists. Likewise there is also no scientific evidence that meaning exists. Both are based on subjective experience and are only what they are experienced to be. Ironically, most of us can accept the presence of scientifically unproven pain much more readily than we can accept the presence of scientifically unprovable meaning.

But the experience of meaning exists as surely as does the experience of pain. A sense of purpose cannot be given by a parent, priest, scientist or therapist. We can be inspired by others, we can be helped toward self-acceptance, but no one can make life seem significant for us by means of subtle argument or moral exhortation. We can only grope toward what we consider the personal task and purpose of any given situation and be open to the meanings that emerge.

Religious and Nonreligious Pathways Toward Meaning

The search can often be easier for those who hold religious belief. A faith that the universe is comprised of one "grand design" provides a comforting framework in which to seek purpose and meaning. From the viewpoint of such a universal concept, nothing can be in vain. "For the joy that was before him, Jesus endured the cross." His disciples portray Christ as willing to endure one of the most painful of all experiences, as someone who believed in a purpose and a meaning beyond his personal suffering. Danger and crisis can even intensify belief. Hölderlin, a religious poet, writes: "Near us yet hard to grasp is the God; where there is peril, there too the deliverer grows." Everything has meaning when perceived through the eye of faith. But what of the nonbelievers? Are those of us who do not subscribe to church ritual or religious doctrine condemned to a state of meaninglessness? For us the search may be different and more lonely, but it is not at all uncommon for nonreligious cancer patients and their families to experience purpose, transcendence and intense personal meaning both in themselves and in their relationships to others. Acts of human service and a growing faith in personal experience (the *doing* and the *being*) can provide great value for those with and without traditional religious belief. The many opportunities are available to all of us.

The search for meaning can be both the most difficult and the most rewarding endeavor of the cancer crisis. In my work with cancer patients, I frequently emphasize its importance and have found that the emphasis often evokes antagonism. Some patients have understandably responded by saying: "If it's so goddamned meaningful, take my place and try it for a while." The point is well taken. Significance varies with the individual who experiences it; that which is a source of meaning to one patient may well be at odds with the needs and tasks of others. However, a great many patients and families have evolved personal meaning from the cancer crisis, and these meanings consistently become their most sustaining sources of strength. It therefore seems appropriate and perhaps essential to explore fully the forms in which meaning can emerge.[2]

Cancer treatment promotes a feeling of greatest urgency. The concept of "lifetime" begins to shrink. Attention shifts to the immediate future. The thought of fulfilling all one's needs, the idea of completing all the unrealized projects of a lifetime can be overwhelming. A sense of life's inherent meaning, for most people cannot be attained through voluminous achievement. Most select one task or embrace one dream that comes to stand for all the others. But, when approached with honesty and commitment, one dream pursued can furnish a sustaining purpose, one task fulfilled can bring a wealth of value into our lives. "The height of a mountain range is not given by the height of some valley but by that of the tallest peak. In life, too, the peaks decide the meaningfulness of the life and a single moment can retroactively flood an entire life with meaning."[3]

Experiences of God are often reawakened during the cancer crisis. The following presentations of these religious experiences will add little to the understanding of those who hold genuine personal faith. But I have worked with many families and health professionals who were confused by a patient's religious interpretation of experience. They did not know how to respond, became antagonistic and thereby failed to appreciate the importance of religious belief as a pathway into a meaningful sense of life. Chapter Thirteen provides an excellent opportunity for those of us who are not religious to gain an understanding of these intense religious experiences. The concepts are a familiar part of the cancer crisis and are so frequently reported by patients and their families precisely because they provide a bridge to the deeper and more meaningful aspects of our lives.

Chapters Fourteen and Fifteen will present a similar search for meaning in nonreligious terms. I have begun with religious belief because it is the most culturally accessible context in which to experience the larger questions of meaning. A clergyman[4] explains this perspective:

Religion can often give people the framework with which to talk about their deeper feelings of life. Many non-religious people do not have a language for expressing these thoughts and feelings, they don't have the necessary symbols. In general, those who have taken the time to explore the meanings of their life are in a less vulnerable position during a crisis, they have already done some rehearsing of concepts and words. But there are relatively few people who pursue the study of philosophy or seriously explore the deeper issues of psychology. There are, however, many who have a heritage of religious training which gives them a language, a container in which to carry their thoughts and feelings.

13

God and Religious Belief

God, whose law it is that he who learns must suffer. Even
in our sleep pain that cannot forget falls drop by drop
upon our heart. And in our own despite, against our will,
comes wisdom to us by the awful grace of God.

—AESCHYLUS

The Reverend Walter E. Johnson[1] is the chaplain of Peninsula General Hospital in northern California. He has been attending the emotional, spiritual and family needs of patients, doctors, nurses, janitors, volunteers and almost everyone else at this medical facility for over twelve years. In the course of one day, I have seen him counseling families, sharing off-color stories, crying with the bereaved, hugging the distraught and praying with the many who request his spiritual solace. This hospital community is his congregation and he is its sensitive and compassionate comforter. I have rarely met anyone who lives the life of religious calling with more dedication to those who suffer. I know him well and have great respect for his therapeutic abilities, and yet to spend time with him is to become increasingly aware that he brings more than sensitivity and counseling skill to his special congregation. To stand by a bed and see a patient begin to weep softly as he prays out loud is to experience another dimension of human assistance—a dimension that rests upon a shared religious belief.

"My work is based on my belief that God resides deep within all of us; the belief that anyone who is willing to go deep into themselves has come into God's presence whether they use the word God or not. I no longer have a concept of God out there. To me, the words 'God' and 'soul' are a shorthand code for talking about the deeper aspects of human existence. The language of God has importance only as it provides contact with these core experiences and with our ability to share them. But the language of God and the role of chaplain contain some distinctive advantages. They provide a framework within which I can establish an intimate contact with others. As a clergyman, I also have permission to hold people, to hug and comfort them, to join hands and to join with families. And, at times, I can use prayer as a way of giving voice to their deep feelings, to their yearnings and fears. When I pray, I try to give a sense of confirmation by introducing the deepest level of previous conversations. My prayers are always a form of acceptance; even when a person feels broken, that feeling can be expressed and the fragments can be woven back into a prayer of wholeness and affirmation. Even when doubt, hatred and guilt torment a patient or family member the prayer can be accepting of such experience and then reach ahead toward resolution. I do not ask God to solve a problem, I never use Him in a passive way. Rather, I pray to God's spirit in that person to help him find clarity and decisiveness and the courage to act. I ask the person to assume responsibility and I sometimes ask it indirectly through a prayer. I ask God to bear witness, and I also use the ancient authority of scripture to affirm a patient's experience when the person adheres to some traditional faith. In fact, the Bible is a kind of collective unconscious that can offer enormous spiritual support by literally affirming all of our experiences. A sense of being among a community of believers also provides an important feeling of belonging."

There are many aspects of the cancer experience that touch upon religious belief. I have chosen three for our consideration. Each contains an inner conflict capable of resolution through religious faith, and each contains the potential for providing new awareness of life's meaning.

Self-Condemnation and Self-Acceptance

Many of us afflict ourselves with an additional burden during the cancer crisis—the condemnation of our experience. We feel *frightened* and accuse ourselves of cowardice; we feel *preoccupied* and accuse ourselves of petty self-indulgence; we feel *doubt* and accuse ourselves of weakness. These common accusations lead to guilt and disillusionment, which are themselves condemned in an endless cycle of self-persecution. The devoutly religious are often the most susceptible to these self-condemnations. An extreme example would be those who equate purity of religious devotion with good health, that is, "If I am good or have enough faith, I will not get sick." This childlike equation is a precarious self-deception and must lead to resounding self-condemnation when we fall ill. Another more subtle version of this equation compels us to interpret fear, despair and defiant anger as a personal failure to accept the will of God. And yet each of us has an inner voice that counsels self-acceptance and opposes these harsh, self-condemning judgments. This voice often echoes scripture, and it is precisely here, amidst these conflicting forces, that the perspective and authority of religious belief offers a pathway toward self-affirmation.

Reverend Johnson addresses himself to this issue:

"I have a deep faith in God that frees me *to* my humanness, it does not free me *from* it. When I use the Bible, when I speak of Christ, I use his humanness as a way of approaching our inner world. This concept fits perfectly with those of the rabbis and Catholic priests with whom I work. It fits for any religious person who is not bound by rigid dogma; it fits for anyone who experiences God as a part of themselves. Imagine a man who is undergoing cancer treatment, who is terrified and angry, who feels ashamed, abandoned and hopeless, who fears he has lost his bearings. Are these experiences different than those of Christ? Remember the garden of Gethsemane when Christ wanted to live so badly he prayed over and over again: 'Let this cup pass from me, this cup of death. . . .' There were waves of doubt and despair followed by waves of acceptance, 'Nevertheless, not my will but thine be done.' Great turmoil and despair were clearly a part of His experience. The Seven Last Words of Jesus demonstrate his deep humanness, touching the most human of concerns for family, physical pain, disillusionment, despair, and only then, of deep acceptance. For example, Jesus needs to know that some loving person will care for his mother and he says: 'John, behold your mother. Mother, behold your son.' The humanness of his pain and continuing physical need are clear when he cries out: 'I thirst, I thirst.' Then He experiences a wave of emptiness and meaninglessness, an anguish familiar to many of us, and He cries out in despair: 'My God, My God, why hast thou forsaken me?' If Jesus can utter these feelings of despair, if Jesus himself can shake his fist against the universe, against the emptiness and doubt and pain, how can any of us dare to condemn ourselves for experiencing the same emotions? It was these very feelings of despair that brought him final acceptance: 'Into Thy hands I commend my spirit.'

"The same themes are found in the psalms of the Old Testament. Most people are familiar with the serene self-acceptance of the twenty-third: 'The Lord is my shepherd, I shall not want. . . . Though I walk through the valley of the shadow of death, I will fear no evil. . . . Surely goodness and mercy shall follow me all the days of my life; and I will dwell in the house of the Lord for ever.' But to read only the twenty-third psalm is to begin at the end. The serenity of the twenty-third comes only after the turbulent despair of the twenty-second: 'My God, my God, why hast thou forsaken me? why art thou so far from helping me, and from the words of my roaring? . . . I cry in the daytime, but thou hearest not. . . . I am poured out like water, and all my bones are out of joint: my heart is like wax; it is melted in the midst of my bowels. My strength is dried up . . . and thou hast brought me into the dust of death.' It is a psalm of utter despair and it must precede the affirmation and acceptance of the twenty-third which follows.

"Whenever I work with people who are angry, disillusioned, hopeless and despairing, I encourage them to drop further and further down into their pain. I do not want them to cheer up. I try to encourage their tolerance of deeper despair because I am confi-

dent that they will touch bottom and that self-acceptance and serenity will then begin to break through. Over and over again, the
wisdom of scripture brings us to our humanness, not away from it,
to the acceptance of our imperfection and to an affirmation of the
light and dark of our wholeness.

"I remember one patient who was in one of the blackest depressions I had ever seen. Alex was a religious man with a deeply
religious background. He had been extremely successful in his career but following his cancer treatment he had fallen into physical
exhaustion and despair. His treatment was successful but the despair
and fatigue continued unabated. I asked him what he saw when he
looked inside himself and he replied, 'Blackness, pitch-black emptiness.' We spent a good deal of time exploring the blackness, discussing the futility and meaninglessness of his life. The despair seemed
to get only blacker. I encouraged him to go farther but I was worried. I had never worked with anyone quite so despondent. As we
talked I recalled a verse which expressed similar emotions and we
read the seventy-seventh psalm together. '. . . My sore ran in the
night, and ceased not: my soul refused to be comforted. . . . Thou
holdest mine eyes waking: I am so troubled that I cannot speak.
. . . Hath God forgotten to be gracious? hath he in anger shut up
his tender mercies?' The psalm is a powerful description of someone
in immense distress: unable to sleep or eat, unable to be comforted
by deeds of the past, feeling utterly abandoned by God. And at that
point Alex looked up and said with great feeling: 'I thought I was
the only one.' The emotional concurrence with a Biblical figure who
had experienced the same despair became a magnetic bond for him.
He began to talk about not being able to eat or sleep, about those
physical symptoms that prevented his recovery, about his sorrow at
being so abandoned. It was a small but real beginning. I asked him
to look inside again and he replied, 'I still see blackness but I must
admit there are a few spots of light.' When Alex felt a bonding with
another person of religious authority, he was no longer alone and
could experience a growing feeling of hope."[2]

The Biblical portraits of doubt, defiance, anger, disillusionment,
abandonment and fear are as common as the biblical expressions of

faith, peaceful serenity and transcendent joy. Possibilities for deeply enriching experience unfold when religious belief is used to validate the full range of our humanity, when scripture supports our striving toward self-acceptance, when clergymen such as Reverend Johnson help us toward wholeness and beyond the barriers of self-condemnation.

Chaos and the Grand Design

It is hard to imagine a more terrifying vision than that which sees the world as existing without order or reason, a place in which we are nothing more than ephemeral creatures who endure for a flickering, meaningless moment and then disappear forever. An unknowable, unforeseeable, unaccountable world affording us neither safety nor comfort, allowing us no possibility of influencing its course! Such a vision confronts us with the idea of an amoral universe and compels us to consider an image so repugnant few of us would wish to entertain it. But the diagnosis of cancer can touch these dark intimations and in doing so intensify our need for a strong belief in some system of order, reason, justice, protection and meaning. Genuine religious belief can fulfill this need and those of us who hold such faith are extraordinarily fortunate.

A belief in God includes the comforting belief in universal order and a grand design. It is a system of belief in which every occurrence has meaning whether fully understood or not. And, for many people, it implies a transpersonal view of the universe which envisions the consummation of perfect justice as an ultimate goal. A vision of transcendent design was expressed succinctly by Einstein when he said: "I cannot believe God played dice with the universe." This belief is a powerful sustaining force, whether God is perceived as an impersonal force or as a conscious personality. There is, however, an added degree of reassurance when God is experienced as a paternal figure perpetually keeping watch over us. The belief that he knows, acknowledges and understands our suffering provides a satisfying feeling of recognition. No experience can be utterly in vain if it is known and understood by a compassionate and powerful father.

A personal God also exists as a vivid presence to whom one can turn; appeals can be made, blame can be vented. An accessible God allows one the freedom to bargain, reason and appeal for an end to anarchy and irrationality. Consider Abraham's audacious confrontation with God when He threatened to destroy Sodom and Gomorrah.[3] Abraham stood before the Lord and scolded Him: "Peradventure there be fifty righteous within the city: wilt thou also destroy and not spare the place for the fifty righteous that are therein? That be far from thee to do . . . to slay the righteous with the wicked. . . . Shall not the Judge of all the earth do right?" After some brief deliberation, God agreed. He would spare the city if there were fifty righteous men. But Abraham continued: "Wilt thou destroy the city for lack of five?" And God again relented: "If I find there forty and five, I will not destroy it." Abraham pushed for forty and God said: "I will not do it for forty's sake." Begging the Lord's permission, he appealed for thirty and then twenty and then three. God gave his final verdict: "I will not destroy it for ten's sake." Here is a remarkable religious phenomenon—a mortal man reasoning with a just God who has absolute power over life and death. It is an incredibly reassuring image. A reasonable, accessible, all-powerful father who watches over us, gives meaning to our actions, judges us fairly and maintains the moral order of the universe. Belief in such a God can surely dispel the terrifying vision of chaos associated with the cancer crisis. The force of this belief is well illustrated by the following story of Hally and Greg:

"We lived in a very small town in Virginia, all of us, and we belonged to a prayer fellowship which was an important part of our lives. Greg quit his job when it began to require his traveling away from home for long periods of time and tried to find a small business. One after another seemed promising but didn't work out, and then this wonderful opportunity came up in California. We were very excited and moved right out. Within the first four months that we were here, not knowing anyone, not having any church group, feeling completely alone, it turned out that Greg had cancer. We were in desperate straits and I just could not conceive of what would become of me should he die. We turned to our faith in God and He brought us through. I began to think: would God have brought us all the way to California after all those false leads, simply to have Greg die of cancer before we could get started? It didn't seem possible. And another part of it involved our daughter. Susan, who had been in Canada trying to start a career, was having a great deal of frustration and little success. She had come home just the week before Greg's illness was diagnosed. And I began to think: would God have brought her home to help keep the new business going during Greg's treatment if he were not going to recover and take over again? That didn't seem possible either. It all seemed a part of some design and the design led to the fact that he would live, that this would be a new beginning for us. That belief, the certainty that all of these things were a message that said he will live, that certainty kept me going."

Greg had his surgery, built up his new business, and they began their new beginning. But, during the time of doubt and dark unknowing, their belief in a universal design, orchestrated by a kind father, was what "carried them through." The experience had lasting effect. "Our lives are deeper now and each day seems to have a precious quality that we are eternally grateful for and see as God's blessing and God's benevolence to us."[4]

Hally experienced the presence of an underlying design to the universe, a unifying system encompassed by God's awareness. The cancer crisis seems to inspire such deep intuitions. For some, like Hally, they are felt in religious terms; for others, the experience is less defined, areligious and highly personal. The deep subjective *experience* of universal order and meaning cannot be expressed in the language of logic. But it is certainly available to many people who go through such periods of stress.

Armed Resistance and Peaceful Surrender

Hally believes that she has always submitted to God's will and is grateful for her family's precious life together. But for many of us the surrender to powerful forces acting upon our lives is in violent conflict with our defiant fighting instincts. It is not at all uncommon to want to give oneself over, to trust in one's fate, to surrender control and responsibility and then a short time later to reverse oneself and want to fight, while yet again, still later, to return to a desire for release and passive acceptance. The *resistance-surrender* cycle is profoundly human. One woman expressed the conflict with poignant clarity: "I have cancer and I have to overcome it. I want to overcome it very badly. [But] sometimes when I'm in pain, I feel like . . . why can't I just wake up dead? That's a very funny thing to say. Why can't I wake up dead."[5] It is a paradoxical emotion and yet it captures the ambivalence perfectly; I want to surrender (in this case to die) *and* I want to wake up triumphant.

A dynamic life contains both the inner force of heroic resistance and the inner force of acceptance and surrender. When we feel beaten, we would do well to reach for our fighting spirit, and when we find ourselves unproductively thrashing against an irreversible reality, we would profit from a greater ability to surrender and accept it. The crucial judgment rests upon an intuitive understanding of when fighting is appropriate and when surrender seems the wisest course. The well-known prayer of St. Francis speaks of this understanding: "Oh God, grant me the serenity to accept the things I cannot change, the courage to change the things I can and the wisdom to know the difference." The appeal is for the clarity to make such a judgment and for the courage to enact the chosen course. It is a remarkable, life-affirming prayer that speaks directly to the struggle between resistance and surrender.

This struggle is present to some degree in all of us, especially during times of stress. A quite different example of the same resistance-surrender conflict often occurs during cancer treatment. Many of us fight the therapeutic procedures at every turn, for they can seem as assaultive as the cancer itself. We do so despite the fact that we know they are attempts to save our lives. In the following instance, the ambivalence was resolved by means of an astonishing religious surrender.

"Sarah is a fighter, a dynamic and religious woman, a well-known community leader involved in a disappointing marriage. She had a wild love affair for a number of years with a prominent lawyer who suddenly died of cancer, and she went through a painfully extended period of secret, guilt-ridden grief. Two years later Sarah herself had to undergo critical surgery. She became tremendously tense prior to her operation—terrified of being made unconscious, of being vulnerable to a surgeon, of dying. But primarily of being out of control. This was one of her lifelong themes. She had always fought to stay in control. As we spoke of these fears, especially her compulsion to manage everything, I began to wonder what *letting go* meant to her. I said: 'I am going to mention a word. Tell me what ideas come to mind.' And then I said *surrender*. She talked about confusion, about crying, about being lost; all associations to the word *surrender* were negative and frightening.

"I asked her to think of a situation in which surrender might seem appropriate. She thought for a long time and then talked about surrender in love. Warren had been a strong, dynamic man and she had been able to surrender herself to him. She could never do so with her weak husband but was able to with this man whom she had loved so much. We talked about how much joy her ability to surrender to love had given her. I asked her if it was possible to think of the experience of surgery in terms of surrendering some of her control to those who were caring for her. At first she was confused, but the image began to grow, and as she spoke she kept moving her hands outward, with the palms up and receptive. I asked her to notice her hands and she said: 'It looks like I'm offering myself, it seems like a peace offering.' Sarah began to develop and embellish the image: 'I can see myself going down to surgery. They are wheeling me in and they are laying me out on a table. It seems like an altar. I'm surrounded by people who care for me, who are here to help me, who are laying healing hands on me. There is a large light in the operating theater and it is like the light of God. I know it's just a physical light but I'll open up to it and God's healing strength will pour into my body. His warm, pure, healing light.' And, as Sarah expanded this image, she became exalted and full of joyful anticipation.

"The surgery was successful and her recovery astonishing. I saw her the evening after the operation and, even though she had just had major surgery, she seemed to glow. She described the entire process as a monumental spiritual undertaking, as a turning point in her life."[6]

We can see from the preceding accounts that genuine religious belief is capable of furnishing a sustaining strength and providing deeply meaningful experience during the cancer crisis. If we can appreciate its important role in the adjustment to serious illness and the possibility of death, we will find ourselves less puzzled and confused by what is often the sudden awakening of religious sensitivity and intense emotion in cancer patients and their families. Belief in God and the authority of scripture can further self-acceptance and the ability to withstand the cruel blows of self-condemnation. It may rescue us, patient and relative alike, from the terror of chaos and help us resolve the universal conflict between armed resistance and peaceful surrender. There can be no doubt that the idea of God provides enormous comfort and meaning for those who are fortunate enough to believe. But similar experiences are available to any of us, with or without belief in God. One of the most meaningful endeavors involves the offering of service to those in need.

14

Acts of Human Service

> A farmer must know the fence which bounds his land but
> need not spend his life standing there, looking out, beat-
> ing his fists on the rails; better he till his soil, think of
> what to grow, where to plant the fruit trees. However
> small the area of freedom, attention and devotion may
> expand it to occupy the whole of life
> —ALLEN WHEELIS, *How People Change*

The search for meaning contains a fundamental polarity: two conflicting aspirations that often cause confusion and distress. One pro-
pelling force within us strives toward uniqueness, seeking to make
each of us distinguishable from all others. In the grip of the polar
force we yearn to be in harmony with others, absorbed into the
world that surrounds us. We want to be unique *and* we want to be
at one with the flow of life. All of us experience the struggle to some
degree; many of us seek its resolution.

The Quest for Immortality

The two polar aspirations emerge during the cancer crisis. On the
one hand, we want to be recognized and to have our life stand for
something purposeful: to drop at least one significant pebble into the
water, to make by intention one discernible ripple. Although we can

never be sure whether our work, children or acts of human service will produce lasting impact, we want to perform those tasks that carry some measure of unique significance and hold some promise of remembrance. These, our most purposeful acts, seem larger than the random occurrences and experiences of our everyday lives. To aspire toward uniqueness is to aspire toward immortality. And yet the emotional forces pulling us toward harmony with our surroundings are also an aspiration toward immortality. To be a part of the universe—this too is to be immortal. The conflicting aspirations are not incompatible.

As a twelve-year-old boy, I drove my father to distraction: "I've done nothing with my life," I'd complain. "I'll have no adventures or achievements, no stories to tell my grandchildren." I seriously believed that there was nothing distinctive about me, nothing that could possibly survive and be remembered. The distress seems childish but the suffering was real. I can still recall the sixth-grade science class in which I resolved my dilemma. We were learning that the stars we saw in the night sky might well not exist. Since the light took millions of years to reach us, the star might well have burned out or exploded, while we could still behold the light that had left its surface millions of years before. My excitement and relief were indescribable. I walked about in deep reverie, imagining the light reflecting off our planet and carrying *my* image toward the stars. I walked in open fields and imagined that a million years after the death of my great-grandchildren (with or without tales of my heroic deeds), my light image could still be seen by those with powerful telescopes in far-off galaxies.

These child's musings reveal a premature but universal yearning for immortality. Those of us with strong traditional belief hope for resurrection, but the desire for immortality may assume other forms as well. It is possible to strive beyond one's immediate needs and to experience a larger world of meaning by offering a valued part of oneself to others and thereby contribute to their well-being. The act of giving the best of oneself is often experienced as a fulfillment of the universal quest for immortality. Those who honor such offerings step beyond themselves, are recognized and remembered; they ex-

perience their lives as distinctive and purposeful. They agree with
Einstein, who wrote: "Only a life lived for others is worthwhile."

Meaning Through Service

Charlotte was a highly respected instructor at a nursing college
when she was told that she had incurable cancer. She continued her
work until forced by weakness to become a patient. During the
months that followed she began to experience the isolation that she
had heard so many other cancer patients describe. As her condition
worsened even colleagues and students began to stay away from her.
Charlotte's sense of loss was extreme. She felt a sense of lonely
desolation and asked for a tape recorder so that she might describe
the experience of hospitalized dying for young nursing students. She
hoped to make her personal experience more understandable and
less frightening to them. However, her request was denied by the
staff and her family because they felt it would make her too "morbid."[1] There is no way of knowing how valuable this woman's
account might have been for the purpose of instruction. But there
is no question that the recordings would have brought a profound
sense of meaning into *her* life. The loss of the work and relationships
she valued more than anything else in life could have been transformed into a meaningful account that would have become a part of
her life's work. It is a tragedy and an outrage that her life was denied
this increment of meaning.

The experience of loss often inspires an attempt to repossess what
has been lost; these attempts contain potential meaning and possible
service. Following the death of a loving mother, who had sustained
him for many years, Proust dedicated himself to a serious undertaking for the first time in his life. He gave profound meaning to the
remaining years of his life by writing *Remembrance of Things Past* and
seeking to retrieve in imagination what was lost to him in reality.
This creative endeavor became his life's work and eventually established him as an international literary figure.

We are, each of us, capable of deriving a sense of purpose from our loss and of making this devastating experience a means for worthwhile action. Offers of human service are always possible and may redeem our darkest hour.

It is impossible to know when opportunities for meaningful acts will occur. Frankl[2] tells the story of a man sentenced to life imprisonment on Devil's Island. A fire broke out during the boat trip to prison. Released from his handcuffs, the convict voluntarily saved the lives of ten people and was pardoned for this act of heroism. But let us consider his despair prior to this event. He could not know that he was about to be given the opportunity to reclaim his life as he stood on the dock, a doomed convict heading for exile. None of us can ever be sure that there are no further possibilities for meaning in our life. Acts of human service await us, requiring only our attention and commitment.

I could not cite a more dramatic instance of the potential for life-sustaining meaning through acts of human service than the events that took place in an English mental hospital during the bombing raids of World War II. The inmates of this ward were "catatonic schizophrenics," who required total care and had been hopelessly withdrawn from reality, often for periods of many years. When it became necessary to use the ward to house the wounded and it was obvious that there were not enough volunteers to attend them, the mental patients voluntarily began to nurse the injured. The psychiatric patients became alert and active; many who had been silent for years even began to speak. However, as soon as the war had ended, as soon as the opportunities for service had disappeared, almost all sank back into their former state of helpless, mute withdrawal.[3]

Offers of Personal Experience

There are an infinite number of services capable of providing a sense of personal significance. Many are efforts to prevent others from knowing the same distress that one has personally suffered. The entertainer Nanette Fabray, afflicted with hearing loss from childhood, was an active promoter of programs to aid the deaf. Her husband died after nineteen years of marriage and she learned the hardships faced by widows and widowers: "Do you know that one out of every four widows is broke a year after the death of their husband? I couldn't have imagined what would happen to me or how unjust the laws are. Now I know how much needs to be changed." She became involved in a movement dedicated to changing those laws. This woman responded to the experience of two catastrophic losses in precisely the same way. She became active in efforts to alleviate the conditions of those in similar distress: "It's very simple, I don't want others to have to go through what I did."[4]

Nelson Shields, the father of a boy senselessly killed in one of the San Francisco "Zebra" murders, joined a citizens' lobby, became its executive director and launched a national campaign to ban handguns. After his son's death, he was tormented by the question: "Why my son?" He tried going back to religion but could find no meaningful answer there. He then decided that the only way he could make sense out of the "random madness that had extinguished a bright light" was "to do something more meaningful than continuing to chase the almighty buck." This bereaved father elected to make his mission the banning of all handguns. As he says: "I've never been involved in this kind of activity . . . but I see no reason why handguns should be in civilian hands. The only purpose a handgun has is to kill people." He hopes to prevent other fathers from experiencing the same tragic loss by destroying all pistols in the United States.[5]

There are thousands of acts of human service that have emerged from the experiences of the cancer crisis. Many are associated with organizations, many are simple individual responses: Wilma King could not chew following her surgery. She discovered that there were no liquid-diet recipes available, began experimenting and compiled recipes for the best of her blended meals in a modestly priced book entitled *Blend and Mend.* It contains specific caloric content for each recipe and even has salt-free diets. Her book has been extremely helpful to many patients, and the process of creation was understandably meaningful to Wilma King.[6]

Terese Lasser had a radical mastectomy many years ago. She suffered post-surgical problems comparable to those of many other women, but unlike those who preceded her, she dedicated herself to the founding of a national volunteer visiting organization, which she named Reach to Recovery. "Reaching, for that is the key—the physical reaching that gave me back strength and confidence in my body. And the spiritual reaching out to others, to life. In helping others, I helped myself."[7] Thousands of women are now helping one another through the Reach to Recovery program.

Dr. Richard Wolk and his wife, Pat, felt isolated when their son was dying of leukemia and were outraged that so few national funds were being spent on cancer research. They helped found the organization called Candlelighters and launched a variety of local and national activities. At one crucial juncture the Candlelighters collected over fifteen thousand signatures in less than two weeks. When the National Cancer Act was passed by Congress in 1971, the Candlelighters were recognized as a significant factor in achieving its passage.[8] This organization has continued to grow and provide an emotional refuge for parents of seriously ill children.

There are thousands and thousands of former cancer patients and family members who derive a great deal of meaning from donating their services to volunteer visiting organizations. Some, like those in the Candlelighters, are parents who continue to work-through their feelings of loss: "I helped another mother whose daughter was dying, not long after our son died . . . you know, it was like losing him again and I was able to make peace with some of the feelings. People looked at me and thought, here she is, she's just lost her son and she's working with this girl that's dying. People were afraid to talk to me; they believed I'd really gone off the deep end. But that time and that work saved me." A father says: "Shortly after our daughter died I could really feel that by doing things for other people I was sorting myself out. It was almost tangible to me. That feeling began to go after a while and today I'm not sure why I'm still visiting other parents. But I imagine that it's the same thing going on; I'm just not quite so aware of it."[9]

Some cancer patients feel lucky to be alive and welcome the opportunity to repay a debt: "I've had cancer and so I feel . . . it's hard to explain. In the past I've knocked on doors for mental health groups (who knows, I might need it someday) and for the Heart Association and all the rest of it. But now it's pretty much just the Cancer Society. It seems like the opposite of 'I might need it some day.' I did need it and now I'd like to help."[10]

Former cancer patients and family members often visit others because they feel that they have a special kind of knowledge and competence to offer. They feel that they've earned their "credentials" by having gone through the cancer experience: "I like to be doing something I know about. Having had it, I feel comfortable talking to others. If I could be a psychologist that would be great but I'm not and never was. In this niche in Reach to Recovery, I feel qualified and know that I can help people."[11] This woman did not allow cancer treatment to diminish her self-esteem. Rather, she used her experience to increase the competence and personal authority with which she regards herself. She is absolutely correct in doing so. No psychologist, physician, social worker, nurse or clergyman in the world knows more about the experience of cancer than does a cancer patient. This former patient makes a valid claim to her knowledge honestly acquired and rightfully asserts the meaning her visits bring to her and others.

Many patients and family members are still furious about abuses they experienced at the hands of an impersonal hospital system. These "veterans" want to offer their knowledge and experience; they want to guide and protect others from similar mistreatment: "A lot has to do with this business of how horrible the whole situation was, with the fact that you know what it's all about. I feel an obligation. I've learned so much and I hate to drop the ball. I'd hate to leave a family at the mercy of those people."[12]

Acts of human service do not have to be tied to the cancer experience in order to give one's life a sense of purpose. One woman explains: "I lost my husband almost forty years ago. He died so unexpectedly and quickly of cancer. I could make no sense of it and I was lost. This was the time when they were evacuating Japanese Americans to those camps, whole families at one time. I went with them and they literally saved my life because they needed me.

. . . I was a nurse and I felt just like them, for I too had lost everything, but I could help them by being a nurse and slowly the pain began to go away."[13]

A Gift to One's Family

Another shade of meaning grows out of acts of service performed for one's family and friends. The depth of personal significance provided by illness may even be felt entirely in symbolic terms. Several years ago, a woman with a family of six was watching a television program on health. She heard and never forgot the statistic that one of every six people will eventually have cancer. She mistakenly took the information literally and fervently prayed that she, among her family of six, would be stricken. When, years later, a lump in her breast was diagnosed as cancer, she felt her prayers had been answered. She experienced no anxiety, rage or depression, nor did she feel any need to grieve. Relief and gratitude were the only emotions she can recall. Since she believed she had been chosen to suffer for her family, the illness with which she was afflicted assumed dimensions of great importance. She felt that she was saving her family from cancer for all time. Two years later, however, widespread cancer was discovered in her husband and he died within a few months. The woman was bewildered. Nothing made sense; her prayers and sacrifices were in vain; their purpose had vanished and she became depressed for the first time. Circumstance had stripped away the meaning of her seemingly purposeful act. Within weeks she began the search for another interpretation of the cancer experience.[14]

The span of our life contains ample room for an infinite variety of human gifts: expressions of love, the perpetuation of cherished values, the enjoyment of precious moments. Even when cancer treatment cannot cure the disease, there is still time to offer a gift of human service. A wife and mother, in the following instance, discovered her unique form of service. Her early life had been one of deprivation and repeated loss. The diagnosis of cancer was experienced as one more assault. Her outrage and ensuing depression were entirely understandable. At first, she dealt with the stress of the cancer experience in a manner consistent with the patterns of both her present and original families. Their primary strategy for dealing with tension, fear and stress consisted of pointed accusation; they attempted to intimidate each other through overbearing hostility. Although she and her husband entered family therapy because of their son's school-related problems, within months the focus of attention had shifted to their marital relationship and the meaning of her illness. In one important, video-taped session, she was shocked to behold herself as an attacking, abusive and hurtful wife rather than the charming person she had always imagined. She could see that the façade of "strength" with which she had sought to cover her anxiety was blatantly expressed as an intensely alienating rage. The confrontation with her image both shocked and repelled her.

Primary cancer treatment, in this instance, did not arrest her tumor growth. Chemotherapy was begun but also failed to retard the spread of disease. It was very important for her to know when the terminal phase of her illness was occurring, for it was then that she began to struggle with what was for her the central issue of her existence—"the way of living and the way of dying." She felt she needed to use the time that was left to her in some meaningful way but did not at first know how to do so. She shuddered at the image of herself as destructive and began to consider the kind of memory she would like to leave her family. The answers became clear: She wanted to be remembered as a woman who was caring and vital. She wanted to free herself from the emotional burdens she had inherited from her parents. She hoped to alter the pattern of her family's ongoing life, and she wanted to bring into being a more gracious home for the next generation. The last year of her life was dedicated to this task. According to her husband, son and relatives, she completely succeeded. When she died, she asked that a letter be read at her funeral. In this letter, she told her friends to be happy for her because she was no longer in pain. She reassured her husband that, despite their angry fights, she remembered well the many good and happy times. And she described the great pleasure she felt in the kind of person her son had become and how much she hoped he would feel free to live his own life. This woman had accomplished her task. For the first time, a generous, loving spirit had been brought into their family life. She had discovered and fulfilled her life's affirmative service.[15]

A sense of purpose can be derived through acts of human service which occur even after one's death. Some people offer their bodies for scientific research, some offer specific organs for transplantation. Laura cherished her visual perceptions of the world; sight was the most valued of all her faculties. She made arrangements to have her "eyes" transplanted when she knew that she was soon to die. Her doctor announced at her funeral services that the corneal transplant had been successful and that a young boy would now be able to see. The thought of this offer provided a sense of high value to Laura, and the fact of it was also meaningful to her family.[16]

Acts of human service lift one beyond the circumstances of the cancer experience. They are a movement toward life, and it matters little whether they consist of a new undertaking or the revival of an old commitment, whether they involve the deepening of family ties or the initiation of new relationships. Acts of human service all lead toward life and the many possibilities of offering and accepting care. Cancer treatment, like the process of aging, can diminish youthful appeal, sexual attractiveness and some bodily functions. But the capacity to give, to love, to offer one's knowledge and comfort grows with time and experience. Imposed limitations do not destroy one's ability to search for the most purposeful of personal endeavors, and the search almost always proves to be worthwhile.

15

The Faith of Personal Experience

With time we may surprise a trace of footsteps
deep in toil across the measure of our days,
seeding the dawn, and never pausing,
in the midday heat, for barley-water brewed with mint:
Unseen but eager presences, who wish to keep us
from a knowledge of their toil, who would
if we should turn on them with gratitude
step back within that natural world
which shares their ripe and tender thought.
  —KIM CHERNIN, *Treasures of Darkness*

Cultural Prohibitions

The high points of a lifetime are recorded in memory by means of the intense emotion that accompanied them. And yet, for most of us, meaning derived from personal experience seems almost forbidden. Religious faith and acts of human service are encouraged; they are validated and rewarded. But paying tribute to one's personal feelings can often cause conflict and distress. The difficulties of deriving meaning from this source are dramatically demonstrated in the following discussion.[1] Several couples who had lost children because of cancer and a group of former cancer patients discuss their feelings:

DORIS: Compared with you young couples and what you've been through, I'm humbled at the superficiality of what's happened to me.
MARY: What are you talking about? If I ever lost a breast I'd be beside myself.

DORIS: Let's face it, it's not the same (begins to weep). . . . I'm thinking of my child and how horrible it would be. Compared to that, what I've had is nothing, just nothing. I think I've indulged myself so much when it's nothing (weeping).

JANE: I hate to hear you use the words "indulge myself" as if there were something wrong with having feelings.

DORIS: But I know that what these young couples have gone through is much deeper and more tragic than what I went through. It's as if I've been too involved in my own emotions when there are things much more important than yourself. I don't know. . . . I'm sorry, I'm terribly embarrassed.

GROUP: No, no, no.

MARIAN: The pain of my child seemed more important to me than anything I was feeling. It wasn't the dying, it was the pain. I wish I could have taken it from her because I'd have understood it so much better.

MILDRED: I lost my father two years ago and I'd have gladly changed places with him. I had cancer but it wasn't so bad. I can't stand to see people suffer and I'd almost rather take the pain onto myself than see them suffer. This is wrong, I know, but when I saw my dad dying, I wanted to trade places with him. His suffering seemed so much more than my own.

MARIAN: I feel like I indulged myself too. My baby was only six months old. What if someone loses a sixteen-year-old? I think, my God, sixteen years old and then I feel like you do. She was only a baby and I hadn't invested sixteen years of love.

DONALD: Our daughter only lived for six months and during that time a father's involvement is small. I can remember Marian nursing her, getting up at all hours of the night. She was so sick and I was feeling bad and I'd start thinking to myself: "My God, look what she's going through. She's carried the child for nine months, went through all the pain and then all that after she was born." And I would think: "Why should I be feeling so much pain; hers must be so much greater." I was tearing myself apart. Angry one day, sad the next, but feeling I had no right to be feeling so much compared to Marian.

JANE: I can hear my mother saying, "I think you stroke your feelings." . . . I didn't know at first what was making me feel so angry. But it was because I was always being told that I indulged myself, that I should not feel so many things, that I should cover them up.

MARIAN: I thought that chapter was closed, that I was just into caring for the other kids, diapers and all. But I haven't resolved the feelings, I've only buried them. [*What does "resolve" mean to you?*] I don't know because if I ever lost my feelings . . . (bursting into tears) then it would be as if it were all in vain.

There is a theme that permeates this entire conversation. Clearly stated it might read, I have not earned the right to feel what I am feeling. Each person believes that if he had experienced the suffering visited upon another he could then have acknowledged and accepted his own intense emotion. Each person imagines that he would feel justified in what he feels if only he were in someone else's shoes. But the group discussion dramatically reveals that the emotional prohibition remains intact regardless of circumstance. Each group member who accorded others the right to feel denies the same right to himself. Mary, who has lost a son, says: "If I ever lost a breast I'd be beside myself." But Doris responds: "Compared with you young couples and what you've been through, I'm humbled at the superficiality of what's happened to me. . . . Compared to that, what I've had is nothing, just nothing." Others pick up and add variations to the same theme. Mildred says: "I had cancer but it wasn't so bad . . . [Her father's suffering] seemed so much more than my own." Marian says: "The pain of my child seemed more important to me than anything I was feeling." Marian wished desperately to relieve her child from pain. But she dismisses the validity of that highly charged emotion and can only experience the prohibition against feeling. Although Doris has accorded her the right to her feelings ("I know that what these young couples have gone through is much deeper and more tragic than what I went through"), Marian and her husband, Donald, cannot grant it to themselves. Marian says: "I feel I've indulged myself too. My baby was only six months old." Her husband, on the other hand, acknowledges her right to grieve but cannot accept his own feelings. "I was tearing myself apart. Angry one day, sad the next, but feeling I had no right to be feeling so much compared to Marian." Although he was racked with intense feeling, he believed only Marian had the *right* to mourn, and tried to diminish and disown his measure of grief.

The underlying theme of emotional prohibition is clearly stated by Jane as she recalls her mother's rules—don't stroke your feelings, don't indulge yourself, cover your feelings up. And Marian, with a burst of profound intuitive knowledge that defies all prohibition, finally states the forbidden truth: "If I ever lost my feelings . . . then it would be as if it were all in vain."

Each member of the group yearns to be able to accept his feelings as valid. And yet each, although secretly desirous, denies himself the right to do so. For many of us, the most memorable, the most meaningful moments of life occur when we experience surging emotion. To feel anything intensely is to be intensely alive. To know joy, celebration or despair, to weep at the birth of a child or to weep at the death of a loved one—all intense emotion is infused with significance. To be in touch with the emotional core of one's life is to experience directly the undeniable meaning of one's existence. The members of this discussion group are denying to themselves a meaningfulness inherent in their own experience. They long for permission to accept their grief as valid, seek external justification for feeling intensely, despite cultural prohibition, and their effort becomes part of a search for meaning.

Prohibitions against the acceptance of intense emotion are often found among cancer patients and their families. Consider, by contrast, a hypothetical group of artists discussing their responses to the simple events of life. The poet claims that he weeps at the evening sunset, the painter at the sight of a flower, the composer at the touch of a light breeze. Each imagines himself to be the most creatively responsive to the passing events of life. And, most importantly, each is proud of this ability. The right to experience intense emotion is taken for granted. Cancer patients and their families seem to compete for the highly dubious honor of having the least right to feel anything. The group discussion quoted on the previous pages amply demonstrates this tendency, and many of us share this burden of prohibition. But, in condemning personal experience as self-indulgence, we also condemn a large area of our humanity. Unlike service, in which meaning is found through active *doing*, personal experiences provide us with meaning through active *being*.

Experience, by its very nature, is subjective. There are no cosmic laws that determine the absolute validity of one "correct" range of feeling. Emotions are valid simply because they exist; all carry the potential for meaning because they are experienced. Who is to say that the loss of one person or position is less worthy (in terms of felt experience) than the loss of another? There are no objective criteria that possess the authority to invalidate emotion. There are only arbitrary cultural prohibitions and, of course, guilt. Cultural taboos are externally imposed (Jane's mother forbidding her to "indulge herself" by feeling); guilt is internally sanctioned (I am unworthy to feel what I feel). But no one, not even the one who suffers, acts with wisdom when he banishes from his life the meaning carried by intense personal experience.

Emotion as a Source of Meaning

Almost any human emotion can enrich life and make it meaningful. Four months after his cancer treatment, an unusually undemonstrative husband sat down with his wife, took her hand and told her how much he had always loved her. He told her that, although he rarely spoke of such things, he was grateful for the life they had shared together and for everything she had given him. Several months later she said: "I sort of always knew, but I'll never forget my tears of happiness hearing him say it. For one time, he gave up being a hard-headed Swede."[2]

A granddaughter derived immense meaning from a similar experience: Amy had been raised in a family with little love and much neglect. The only person who had ever really cared for her was her grandfather's "new wife," a woman he married when Amy was still an infant. Despite the fact that Grandma Ann never felt accepted by the family, she provided the one warm haven for Amy throughout her childhood. In later years, Amy would take her children for an obligatory visit home each summer. The trips were a meaningless ritual except for their short, wonderful stays with Grandma Ann. When Amy learned that her grandmother had widespread inoperable cancer and would live for only several months, she felt that her "only real home" was being "ripped out" of her life. And, although she was almost paralyzed with grief, she went on one last visit to say goodbye.

Once there, Amy could feel her grandmother's loneliness and recurring doubt. More than anything else Amy wanted to talk about these feelings, but the family cautioned against it. No one, including Grandma Ann, had ever expressed strong emotions and everyone (all family members and the doctors) believed she would only be burdened by them now. But, despite the warnings and despite their family history of spartan behavior, Amy did begin to talk to her about their life. "We had never done so before. You know, a little teasing about how we had always had a crush on each other, but never any serious talk. This time I told her exactly what she had always meant to me. (Tears and soft weeping.) How she had been the only one . . . in my whole childhood . . . who seemed to love me . . . who didn't see me as another stupid, skinny kid. I told her about how lonely I had always been at home, about how eagerly I waited for my visits to see her and how she couldn't possibly be more family; that she was the best part of any family I'd ever known. And she . . . she held my hand and . . . and kept saying how much she loved me . . . what a beautiful little girl I was . . . how much she loved me, and I kept telling her that she never ever was a step-grand-mother but always my only real grandma. . . . I'll hold that moment for the rest of my life—that I could reassure her over and over again . . . make her feel how important she was to me and hear her say how much she loved me."[3]

Amy was able to overcome a well-established family history of emotional denial, and by doing so she brought a profound and highly valued experience into both their lives. Meaning, for each of them, arose directly from an experience in which they acknowl-edged their feelings, accepted them and shared them together.

Accepting the validity of one's emotional experience is certainly not an easy achievement in our culture. However, there are ways to encourage the process of acceptance. An old man I knew had a special method of capturing the essence of his feelings. He had been a lecturer, and he used his verbal facility to give a distinctive impor-tance to his experience of illness. He would imagine himself standing before his students and bestowing upon them the philosophical ramifications of each "important emotion." He was able to give authority to his feelings by creating an imaginary podium for each new sensation and thought. And he was able to give himself the authority to honor these feelings "publicly" by assuming his old professorial stature.

The opportunity to tell one's story can provide a similar liberating context. Important experiences take on recognizable significance during the process of shaping their chronology and pattern. I have often imagined providing a service for seriously ill people by recording significant events and experiences in their lives, making them into a personal chronicle and permitting them to become a part of the family inheritance. The threat to life cannot help but carry a new perspective; new reflections upon oneself and one's life invariably emerge. Meaning emerges when these feelings and thoughts are treated seriously and given a valid place in the course of an illness or death.

I can think of no more beautiful example of an evolving openness to personal experience than the story of Gloria.[4] Not only did her ability to accept and honor her own experience bring new meaning into her life, but her openness brought a transcendent awareness and a compassion for others that will always be remembered by those who knew her. This woman's cancer crisis began with the darkest of personal experiences, but once faced, these dark images were replaced with an intense illumination.

Gloria was fifty-six years old when her physician told her that she had cancer. She had become a success in society—wealthy, well dressed, poised and blessed with unusual social grace. But she was unable to deal with her rampaging anxiety and confusion following the diagnosis of cancer. She described that time as "when I literally went crazy." Gloria went to talk with a hospital chaplain (whom she knew through charity work) in a state of lonely despair and asked him if he could help her find some faith to sustain her now that her world had fallen apart. It is curious that she turned to a religious man, for she had no religious background or training. In fact, she had carefully avoided two areas throughout her adult life: the concept of religion and the idea of death. Although her cancer treatment was successful, the "monster" image of death had now irreversibly entered her thoughts, and she instinctively turned toward a nonexistent religious belief.

Gloria's unusual fear of death could be traced to a vivid childhood memory, an image implanted at the age of eight. Her father was a tyrannical and sometimes cruel man who hated her pet dog. One day he poisoned the animal and threw it into a woodshed. She remembers that the dog, having been given insufficient poison, cried out for several days. Finally there was silence. She begged her father to tell her what had happened but he angrily ignored her pleas. When Gloria stumbled over her pet many weeks later while playing on a hillside, it was a bloated, rotten carcass. There was a tremendous stench and there were thousands of maggots devouring the decaying body: a grotesque image, seen once and never forgotten. From that point on, she never attended a funeral or considered death. But, following her diagnosis of cancer, she was forced to face the possibility of her own death and began searching for some faith that could offset the horrifying image she carried within her.

Gloria wanted religious belief but had no tradition from which to work. She tried reading the Bible but it seemed a collection of meaningless stories unconnected to any of her life experiences. Religious concepts and invocations were meaningless to her. Yet she continued searching for some way of approaching the dark terror within her. For two years, despite her great anxiety and lack of faith, she continued her talks with the hospital chaplain and kept trying to understand her terror. She gradually began to recall events, gradually became capable of describing her experiences of loss, gradually attained an ability to philosophize about life and to at least tolerate her terrifying and unrelenting image of death.

Ten years later, Gloria was rehospitalized with widespread metastatic tumor and she once again asked to speak to the hospital chaplain. He recalled his thoughts and impressions: "I went expecting to see someone devastated by illness and approaching death. Remembering her terror, I expected to see her in a terrible state of despair. But these expectations vanished the moment I entered her room.

She reached out with a warm smile, not the superficial society one I remembered, but a smile of open radiance. The nurse with her also had the same open feeling. With great ease she told me that she wanted to plan her funeral, that she wanted a closed coffin and that she wanted a particular picture placed on top of it. I couldn't help but wonder what meaning the picture carried and so I asked about it. I've never forgotten her answer.

"The picture showed her sitting on a stone wall at the edge of a beautiful lake. It had been taken about a year before our talk. She was ill and in pain and wanted to take one last vacation with her husband. He had fixed up a camper so that she could travel more comfortably and they had come to this mountain lake together. Pain woke her early one morning. Not being able to return to sleep, she dressed and took a walk along the shore. There was a cold stone wall there and she leaned against it, recalling that the coldness of the stones seemed to take away some of the pain. When the rays of the sun emerged over the horizon and began to strike her, she said she felt their warmth penetrate into her body. She said: 'My body opened up and the rays flowed right through me and as the sun warmed me, I began to feel strange, like I belonged to this whole universe whether I lived or died, and at that moment I felt alive in a way I had never felt before in my life.'

"Gloria described how the fear went out of her pain. She said the physical sensations changed completely when the dread disappeared. When she returned home to receive additional treatments, she said people began responding to her in this strange, new, open way. I talked with the nurses in the hospital and they loved her, they just loved her. Several got together and gave her a toy poodle and Gloria told me that, as she received the puppy, full of tears and happiness, she could feel the little heart beating against her hand. She said: 'I could feel the heartbeat growing and growing until I knew that I too was a part of the heartbeat of the universe.' And that same overwhelming feeling of acceptance and peace swept through her again. When I entered her room expecting to find a terrified and devastated patient, I walked into this glowing world of faith born out of her personal experience.

"We talked of many things that day. She spoke of her death: 'I know inside that when I die my love is going to keep vibrating, not just in the hearts of those who know me but in the world itself. That it is a tangible force that will continue on.' I asked if she wanted to hear a similar passage from the Bible. She smiled that smile and I read a portion of II Corinthians, Chapter 5, where St. Paul speaks of death and says: 'So that which is mortal may be swallowed up by life.' This passage touched her for the first time because it reflected *her* experience of life. The sustaining faith she had hoped to find and had never been able to discover in traditional religion had been fully experienced in the deepest part of herself. She nodded as I finished the text and said: 'That's right, that's exactly right.' When she died, her family and friends grieved openly and were comforted by an agreed-upon reality—Gloria had been more alive and happy during the last year of her life than at any other time anyone could remember."

Gloria's profound faith emerged from her intense personal experience. The serenity of her acceptance was preceded by the most dreadful time of terror. Her faith came, in large part, because of her courage and tenacity, because of her readiness to pursue and accept her own emotion. She was willing to acknowledge her anxiety, to explore its origins, to tolerate the terrible fears evoked and to keep searching for a sustaining sense of purpose. Her curiosity was stronger than her fear or self-condemnation.

Numerous personal experiences are destroyed by moral judgments: "I should not be afraid, it's wrong to be depressed, how terrible to be so angry," and so on. These moral pronouncements lead to guilt, which in turn leads to the suppression of what we feel. But feeling, any and all feeling, must be acknowledged and even welcomed if we are to derive from our personal experience the affirming and life-sustaining visions which are an intimate part of our human endowment. Those of us who have been able to build a trusting faith in our experience have had to be open to a wide assortment of intense emotion: terror and repulsion, jealousy, guilt, despair, isolation and frustrated rage. Unfortunately, intense *negative* feelings are almost always the first to be experienced. But to condemn and banish these unwelcome feelings is to deny oneself all the potential meaning that may emerge from the intensity of our personal experience. If a healthy curiosity about these dark emotions can replace the shame and self-condemnation often associated with them, it is possible that we may establish a productive pattern of exploration. Once this shift in attitude has taken place, both dark and joyous experiences can be recognized and acknowledged as a part of the spectrum of human emotion. Amy and Gloria were able to make this shift from self-condemning judgment to self-accepting curiosity, and each derived enormous value from this newly acquired faith in their own experience.

The Validation of Experience

The pursuit of intense experience as a valid source of significance is probably the most arduous pathway toward a deeper sense of life. The validation of personal experience has little social support. The struggle for self-acceptance is frequently interpreted as selfishness or reviled as another shameful manifestation of the "me" decade.[5] Acts of human service are accepted as offerings of help regardless of their deeper motivation. A belief in God carries a universal perspective that transcends personal considerations, and the experience of protectedness so derived is not in conflict with traditional cultural or moral criteria. But achieving a faith of personal experience is quite a different matter.

There is a parallel here to the moral injunctions many of us place on our sexuality. We only enjoy ourselves "with abandon" when swept away by a wave of sexual passion. It is almost as if "something else" or "someone else" had taken over and we did not have to feel responsible for the "shameful" sexual desire. It can be as difficult to accept personal responsibility for grief, fear, despair, joy or anger as for strong sexual feeling. But what would happen if we dared to answer the moral reprimand with a shrug? What might it mean if we replied within ourselves: "Of course I'm responsible for feeling what I feel. I have the right to my experiences and will try to accept all of them. I may not act on all of them but I won't deny their existence. I believe that building a faith in myself is a worthy goal and certainly not a self-indulgence. And I intend to pursue this source of personal meaning." This attitude would mean a great deal even if the tone were tentative. It would be a beginning: a shift from condemnation to attempted validation, from mistrustful vigilance to empathetic curiosity, from being one's worst enemy to becoming an inner ally. It is as decent to be kind and generous to oneself as it is to offer these blessings to another. And if more of us had the courage to pursue a faith in our personal experience, more of us might come to know the unshakable sense of meaning that resides there waiting to be revealed. I can vividly recall a former cancer patient encountering some of the most intensely shameful memories of her childhood. These terrible recollections had always haunted her and more recently had infused her experience of cancer treatment with great alarm. She also had a lifelong habit of dismissing her feelings, but this time she slowly and courageously explored them, overcoming both terror and shame. When I next saw her, she said to me: "I've had this incredible image all week. I see another me, a twin sister of me. She looks very much like I do and she's walking out of the fog. She's waving and smiling at me and walking out of the fog. It has given me such a wonderful feeling."

Are we not, all of us, capable of discovering this radiant being within ourselves and claiming all of our time to live?

Notes

Introduction

1. *The New English-Chinese Dictionary* (Hong Kong: Commercial Press, 1966).

2. Michel de Montaigne, *Selected Essays* (New York: Pocket Books, 1959), p. 23. "So did the Egyptians, who in the midst of their banquetings and in the full of their greatest cheer, cause the anatomy of a dead man to be brought before them."

3. Elisabeth Kübler-Ross, *On Death and Dying* (New York: Macmillan, 1969); Elisabeth Kübler-Ross, *Questions and Answers on Death and Dying* (New York: Collier Books, 1974); Ernst Becker, *The Denial of Death* (New York: The Free Press, 1973); W. Easson, *The Dying Child* (Springfield, Ohio: C. C. Thomas, 1972); Herman Feifel, ed., *The Meaning of Death* (New York: McGraw-Hill, 1959); Marya Mannes, *Last Rights* (New York: Signet, 1975); Mark Pelgrin, *And a Time to Die* (Sausalito: Contact Editions, 1962); L. Pincus, *Death and the Family* (New York: Pantheon Books, 1974); A. D. Weisman, *The Realization of Death* (New York: Jason Aronson, 1974).

Chapter 1: The Dark Cloud of Unknowing

1. *Cancer Facts and Figures* (New York: American Cancer Society Publishers, 1974). The National Cancer Institute defines *cured* as "without evidence of disease five years after diagnosis and treatment."

2. ABC-TV, as recorded in its private survey and reported on its public-affairs program, "I Used to Have Cancer," July 14, 1976.

3. *Cancer Facts and Figures,* 1974.

4. Gallup Organization, Inc., "Women's Attitudes Regarding Breast Cancer," conducted for The American Cancer Society, 1974.

5. San Francisco *Chronicle,* San Francisco *Examiner,* June 19, 1973.

6. L. Fixel, "Coming to This Place." Unpublished poem used with permission of the author.

7. Simone de Beauvoir, *A Very Easy Death* (New York: Warner Books, 1964), p. 24.

8. R. Cantor, personal communications with cancer patients and families and consultations with health professionals working with cancer patients and their families between 1961 and 1977.

9. Ibid.

10. Ibid.

11. J. C. Quint, "The Impact of Mastectomy," *American Journal of Nursing* 63:11 (1963), p. 89.

12. Ibid.

13. Cantor, personal communications.

14. Ibid.

15. E. Goffman, *Stigma* (Englewood Cliffs, N.J.: Prentice-Hall, 1963). *Stigma* is a penetrating discussion of the social consequences that follow a divergence from our cultural norms.

16. Cantor, personal communications.

17. Ibid.

18. Ibid.

19. De Beauvoir, *A Very Easy Death,* p. 37.

20. Cantor, personal communications.

21. Ibid.

22. Ibid.

23. Ibid.

24. V. E. Frankl, *The Doctor and the Soul* (New York: Vintage Books, 1973), p. 94.

25. D. C. Gordon, *Overcoming the Fear of Death* (Baltimore: Penguin Books, 1972), p. 51.

26. Hans Selye, *The Stress of Life* (New York: McGraw-Hill, 1966), p. 128.

27. Cantor, personal communications.

28. Ibid.

29. Ibid.

30. J. Caruthers. As quoted in the San Francisco *Chronicle* on November 14, 1975.

31. Panel discussion, "Helping Your Patients Stage a Comeback from Cancer," *Medical Opinion* (August 1975), p. 12.

32. Gallup, "Women's Attitudes Regarding Breast Cancer."

33. Cantor, personal communications.

34. A. M. Sutherland et al., *The Psychological Impact of Cancer* (New York: American Cancer Society, 1960). Sutherland and his associates published some of the early and significant studies about emotional responses to cancer treatment. Seven classic articles have been collected and republished by the American Cancer Society under the title *The Psychological Impact of Cancer*

and can be ordered from the American Cancer Society, 219 East 42nd Street, New York, New York 10017.

35. W. E. Johnson, Chaplain, Peninsula General Hospital, Millbrae, California. Personal communications between 1974 and 1977.

36. Cantor, personal communications.

37. Sutherland et al., *Psychological Impact of Cancer,* p. 18.

38. Cantor, personal communications.

39. Sutherland et al., *Psychological Impact of Cancer.*

40. Ibid.

41. Cantor, personal communications.

42. Sutherland et al., *Psychological Impact of Cancer.*

43. Cantor, personal communications.

44. Ibid.

45. Susan Martini, unpublished journal. Used with permission of the author.

46. Cantor, personal communications.

47. Ibid.

48. Ibid.

49. Ibid.

50. Sutherland et al., *Psychological Impact of Cancer,* p. 86.

51. C. G. Jung, *Two Essays on Analytic Psychology* (Cleveland: World Publishing Co., 1970).

52. C. G. Jung, *Man and His Symbols* (Garden City, New York: Doubleday, 1968). The quote is referred to by M. L. von Franz in her discussion of individuation, p. 172.

53. W. James, ed., *The Literary Remains of the Late Henry James* (Boston: Osgood Press, 1885), p. 59.

54. News report, KCBS, San Francisco, September 5, 1975.

55. *Cancer in California* 18:1. Published by the American Cancer Society, 1972.

56. V. Richards, *Cancer: The Wayward Cell* (Berkeley: University of California Press, 1972).

57. *Steadman's Medical Dictionary* (Baltimore: Williams & Wilkins, 1972).

58. Heather Parker, age 12, as quoted in the Redwood City *Tribune,* November 1, 1974.

59. Sutherland et al., *Psychological Impact of Cancer,* p. 76.

60. *Cancer Facts and Figures,* 1974.

Chapter 2: Depression and Anger

1. T. J. Craig and M. D. Abeloff, "Psychiatric Symptomatology Among Hospitalized Cancer Patients," *American Journal of Psychiatry* 131:12 (1974), p. 1323; R. D. Rozen et al., "The Psycho-Social Aspects of Maxillofacial

Rehabilitation: Part 1—The Effect of Primary Cancer Treatment," *Journal of Prosthetic Dentistry* 28:4 (1972), p. 426.

2. E. Bibring, "The Mechanism of Depression," in P. Greenacre, ed., *Affective Disorders* (New York: International Universities Press, 1953), p. 34.

3. R. Cantor, personal communications.

4. R. D. Abrams, *Not Alone with Cancer* (Springfield, Ill.: C. C. Thomas, 1974), p. 65.

5. V. McGrath, former director of Befriender Program, Suicide Prevention Program, San Mateo, California. Personal communication.

6. Cantor, personal communications.

7. L. Crammer, *Up from Depression* (New York: Pocket Books, 1972), p. 38.

8. Cantor, personal communications.

9. D. Renshaw, "How Patients and Their Families Cope with Cancer," *Medical Opinion* (August 1975), p. 25.

10. Crammer, *Up from Depression,* p. 8.

11. Sigmund Freud, "Mourning and Melancholia," in Collected Papers, IV (London: Hogarth Press, 1925).

12. Cantor, personal communications.

13. Bibring, "Mechanism of Depression," p. 24.

14. Cantor, personal communications.

15. Ibid.

16. Ibid.

17. A. Rothenberg, "Psychological Problems in Terminal Cancer Management," *Cancer* 14:1063 (1961), p. 1067.

18. Cantor, personal communications.

19. Ibid.

20. Ibid.

21. Ibid.

22. Sutherland et al., *Psychological Impact of Cancer,* p. 25.

23. Cantor, personal communications.

24. Ibid.

25. Ibid.

26. T. Moriarty, "A Nation of Willing Victims," *Psychology Today* (April 1975), p. 46.

27. A. Verwoerdt, "A Communication with the Fatally Ill," *CA—A Cancer Journal for Clinicians* 15:105 (1965); R. H. Dovenmuehle and A. Verwoerdt, "Physical Illness and Depressive Symptomatology," *Journal of Gerontology* 18:260 (1963); and A. Hutschnecker, "Personality Factors in Dying Patients," in Feifel, *Meaning of Death.*

28. L. E. Hinkle and S. Wolff, "A Summary of Experimental Evidence Relating Life Stress to Diabetes Mellitus," *Journal of Mt. Sinai Hospital* 19:537 (1952).

29. E. M. Blumberg, P. M. West, and F. W. Ellis, "A Possible Relationship Between Psychological Factors and Human Cancer," *Psychosomatic Medicine* 16:4 (1954).

30. R. Cantor, "Expression of Anger and Post-Surgical Adjustment," unpublished research completed at the University of California, San Francisco, 1970.

31. A. Wheelis, *How People Change* (New York: Harper & Row, 1973), p. 78.

32. D. Robertson, *Survive the Savage Sea* (New York: Bantam Books, 1974), p. 66.

33. Bibring, "Mechanism of Depression," p. 43.

Chapter 3: The Work of Mourning

1. R. W. White, *The Abnormal Personality* (New York: Ronald Press, 1964), p. 393.

2. Charles Dickens, *Dombey and Son,* as quoted in Gordon, *Overcoming the Fear of Death,* p. 70.

3. Lynn Caine, author of *Widow,* as quoted in an interview in the San Francisco *Chronicle,* June 21, 1974.

4. G. L. Engel, "A Life Setting Conducive to Illness: The Giving-Up/Given-Up Complex," *Annals of Internal Medicine* 69:293 (1968), p. 296.

5. R. Grinker and J. Spiegel, *Men Under Stress* (Philadelphia: Blakiston, 1945).

6. Pincus, *Death and the Family,* p. 12.

7. R. Cantor, personal communications between 1961 and 1977.

8. James Boswell, *Life of Johnson,* ed. by R. W. Chapman and C. B. Tinker (New York: Oxford University Press, 1953), p. 196.

9. Sutherland et al., *Psychological Impact of Cancer,* p. 74.

10. Cantor, personal communications.

11. Kim Chernin, *Mothers and Daughters.* Unpublished manuscript used with permission of the author.

12. P. J. Clayton, "The Effect of Living Alone on Bereavement Symptoms," *American Journal of Psychiatry* 132:2 (1975).

13. Pincus, *Death and the Family,* p. 245.

14. L. H. Schwartz and J. L. Schwartz, *The Psychodynamics of Patient Care* (Englewood Cliffs, New Jersey: Prentice-Hall, 1972); E. Lindemann, "Symptomatology and Management of Acute Grief," *American Journal of Psychology* 101:141 (1944); G. L. Engel, *Psychological Development in Health and Disease* (Philadelphia: W. B. Saunders, 1962); Pincus, *Death and the Family;* and J. Brantner, "Life-Threatening Disease as a Manageable Crisis," *Seminars in Oncology* 1:2 (1974).

15. Kübler-Ross, *On Death and Dying.*

16. V. S. Knapp and H. Hansen, "Helping the Parents of Children with Leukemia," *Social Work* (July 1973).

17. Cantor, personal communications.

18. Ibid.

19. V. Barckley, "Grief, a Part of Living," *Ohio's Health* 20:34 (1968), p. 38.

20. Kübler-Ross, *Questions and Answers on Death and Dying,* p. 98.

Chapter 4: The Politics of Integrity

1. R. W. White, "Strategies of Adaptation: An Attempt at Systematic Description," in G. V. Coelho, D. A. Hamburg, and J. E. Adams, *Coping and Adaptation* (New York: Basic Books, 1974).

2. I want to present Robert W. White's excellent systematic description of adaptation (information, internal organization and autonomy), and I also want to emphasize a somewhat divergent and contradictory point of view. I have therefore chosen to use different names for these children. White's illustrations are based on Murphy's observations, in L. B. Murphy, *The Widening World of Childhood: Paths Toward Mastery* (New York: Basic Books, 1962).

3. W. T. Fitts and I. S. Raudin, "What Philadelphia Physicians Tell Patients with Cancer," *Journal of the American Medical Association* 153:901 (1953); and D. Oken, "What to Tell Cancer Patients," *Journal of the American Medical Association* 175:317 (1961).

4. A. Peck, "Emotional Reactions to Having Cancer," *Cancer* 22:284 (1972); R. D. Abrams, *Not Alone with Cancer* (Springfield: C. C. Thomas, 1974); J. Gunther (interview with F. D. Adair), "Cancer in Our Breast," *Woman's Home Companion* (February 1954); and A. D. Weisman, "The Patient with a Fatal Illness: To Tell or Not to Tell," *Journal of the American Medical Association* 196:201 (1968).

5. Abrams, *Not Alone with Cancer,* p. 42.

6. W. G. Thurman, chairman, "The Child with Cancer," *Proceedings of the American Cancer Society's National Conference on Human Value and Cancer,* Atlanta, June 22, 1972.

7. R. Cantor, personal communications.

8. G. M. Francis, "Cancer: The Emotional Component," *American Journal of Nursing* 69:8 (1969).

9. R. R. Koenig, "Anticipating Death from Cancer—Physician and Patient Attitudes," *Michigan Medicine* 68:17 (1969); and Kübler-Ross, *Questions and Answers on Death and Dying,* p. 55.

10. Peck, "Emotional Reactions."

11. Rothenberg, "Psychological Problems," p. 1071.

12. Abrams, *Not Alone with Cancer,* p. 11.

13. Cantor, personal communications.

14. S. Klagsbrun, "The Psychiatrist's Viewpoint," unpublished case report, 1970.

15. Muhammad Ali, *The Greatest: My Own Story* (New York: Random House, 1975), p. 241.

16. M. L. Fogel and R. H. Rosillo, "Correlation of Psychological Variables and Progress in Physical Rehabilitation," *Diseases of the Nervous System* 30:9 (1969), p. 593.

17. Abrams, *Not Alone with Cancer,* p. 66.

18. H. H. Garner, *Psychosomatic Management of the Patient with Malignancy* (Springfield, Ill.: C. C. Thomas, 1966).

19. Robert Anderson, *After* (New York: Random House, 1974).

20. Ibid.

Chapter 5: Finding the Safe Place

1. Brantner, "Life-Threatening Disease"; Schwartz, *Psychodynamics of Patient Care;* and Abrams, *Not Alone with Cancer.* All of these authors present examples of how professionals often think of delay and denial as merely therapeutic obstacles and then explain their psychological importance.

2. Abrams, *Not Alone with Cancer,* p. 5.

3. Cantor, personal communications.

4. Johnson, personal communications.

5. Abrams, "The Patient with Cancer."

6. Cantor, personal communications.

7. R. D. Abrams and J. E. Finesinger, "Guilt Reactions in Cancer Patients," *Cancer* 6:474 (1953); M. Bard and R. Dyk, "The Psychodynamic Significance of Beliefs Regarding the Cause of Serious Illness," *Psychoanalytic Review* 43:146 (1956); R. Bouchard and N. P. Owens, *Nursing Care of the Cancer Patient* (St. Louis: C. V. Mosby Co., 1972).

8. Sutherland, *Psychological Impact of Cancer,* p. 25; M. F., Bozeman, C. E. Orbach, and A. M. Sutherland, "Psychological Impact of Cancer—Its Treatment," *Cancer* 8:1 (1955).

9. Verwoerdt, "Communication with the Fatally Ill."

10. As quoted in the *Talmud,* Avodah Zarah.

11. Sutherland et al., *Psychological Impact of Cancer,* p. 61.

12. Cantor, personal communications.

13. Bard and Dyk, "Psychodynamic Significance."

14. Cantor, personal communications.

15. Bard and Dyk, "Psychodynamic Significance."

16. D. Ordway, clinical social worker, Head and Neck Cancer Rehabilitation Program, University of California Medical Center, personal communication.

17. Bard and Dyk, "Psychodynamic Significance."

18. Ibid.

19. Abrams, *Not Alone with Cancer,* p. 15.

20. Bard and Dyk, "Psychodynamic Significance."

21. Cantor, personal communications.

22. Sutherland et al., *Psychological Impact of Cancer,* p. 25.

23. Cantor, personal communications.

24. Sutherland et al., *Psychological Impact of Cancer.*

25. Cantor, personal communications.

26. Sutherland et al., *Psychological Impact of Cancer.*

27. Cantor, personal communications.

28. Ibid.

29. Sutherland et al., *Psychological Impact of Cancer.*

30. D. M. Kaplan et al., "Family Mediation of Stress," *Social Work* (July 1973), p. 66.

31. Cantor, personal communications.

32. Pincus, *Death and the Family,* p. 118; J. Hinton, *Dying* (Baltimore: Penguin Books, 1967), p. 181.

33. Anger is another major source of guilt experienced by cancer patients, family members, and friends. It is quite common to want suffering persons to die, to be angry when they continue to "hang on" and to be enormously relieved when they finally "let go." It is also common for patients to be enraged by this impatience. When anger, impatience and relief are declared unacceptable or felt to be too dangerous for expression, they become converted into an oppressive guilt.

34. William Blake, *Illustrations of the Book of Job* (introduction and interpretations by S. Foster Damon) (New York: E. P. Dutton, 1969).

35. Cantor, personal communications.

Chapter 6: The Maintenance of Personal Authority

1. N. Branden, *The Psychology of Self-Esteem* (New York: Bantam Books, 1973), p. 110.

2. R. W. White, *The Abnormal Personality* (New York: Ronald Press, 1964), p. 150.

3. Cantor, personal communications.

4. Ibid.

5. Branden, *Psychology of Self-Esteem,* p. 124.

6. W. James, *The Principles of Psychology* (New York: Holt, Rinehart and Winston, 1890), p. 310.

7. Cantor, personal communications.

8. Gallup Organization, "Women's Attitudes Regarding Breast Cancer."

9. Wheelis, *How People Change,* p. 28.

10. Cantor, personal communications.

11. J. V. Warren, in the panel discussion reported in *Medical Opinion* (August 1975), p. 12.

12. Cantor, personal communications.

13. Ibid.

14. Ibid.

15. Ibid.

16. R. Kushner, *Breast Cancer: A Personal History and an Investigative Report*

(New York: Harcourt Brace Jovanovich, 1976). This excerpt reported in the San Francisco *Chronicle*, March 25, 1976.

17. N. S. Caroline, "Dying in Academe," *The New Physician* (November 1972).

18. Kübler-Ross, *Questions and Answers on Death and Dying*, p. 56.

19. Reach to Recovery Task Force Committee Meetings which I participated in during 1974 and 1975.

20. Abrams, *Not Alone with Cancer*, p. 79.

21. G. J. Annas, *The Rights of Hospital Patients* (New York: Avon Books 1975).

22. "To my family, my physician, my lawyer, my clergyman.

To any medical facility in whose care I happen to be.

To any individual who may become responsible for my health, welfare or affairs:

Death is as much a reality as birth, growth, maturity and old age— it is the one certainty of life. If the time comes when I, ————— —————, can no longer take part in decisions for my own future, let this statement stand as an expression of my wishes while I am still of sound mind.

If the situation should arise in which there is no reasonable expectation of my recovery from physical or mental disability, I request that I be allowed to die and not be kept alive by artificial means or "heroic measures." I do not fear death itself as much as the indignities of deterioration, dependence and hopeless pain. I therefore ask that medication be mercifully administered to me to alleviate suffering even though this may hasten the moment of death.

This request is made after careful consideration. I hope you who care for me will feel morally bound to follow its mandate. I recognize that this appears to place a heavy responsibility upon you, but it is with the intention of relieving you of such responsibility and of placing it upon myself in accordance with my strong convictions that this statement is made."

23. O. C. Simonton and S. Simonton, "Management of the Emotional Aspects of Malignancy," as part of a symposium, New Dimensions of Habilitation for the Handicapped, Florida Department of Health and Rehabilitative Services, June 14, 1974.

24. Dr. Philip M. West as reported in B. Klopfer, "Psychological Variables in Human Cancer," *Journal of Projective Techniques* 21:331 (1957).

25. L. L. LeShan and R. E. Worthington, "Personality as a Factor in the Pathogenesis of Cancer: A Review of the Literature," *British Journal of Medical Psychology* 29 (1956); S. J. Kowal, "Emotions as a Cause of Cancer," *Psychoanalytic Review* 42:3 (1955); F. R. Miller and H. W. Jones, "The Possibility of Precipitating the Leukemic State by Emotional Factors," *Blood*

8:880 (1948); E. P. Pendergrass, "Host Resistance and Other Intangibles in the Treatment of Cancer," *American Journal of Roentgenology* 85:891 (1961); B. Graham, "Psychic and Cellular Aspects of Isolation and Identity Impairment in *Cancer,*" *Annals of New York Academy of Sciences* 164:352 (1969); L. L. Le Shan, "Psychological States as Factors in the Development of Malignant Disease: A Critical Review," *Journal of the National Cancer Institute* 22 (January 1959); C. B. Bahnson, "Psychophysiological Complementarity in Malignancies," *Annals of New York Academy of Sciences* 164 (1969); L. L. Le Shan, "An Emotional Life-History Pattern Associated with Neoplastic Disease," *Annals of New York Academy of Sciences* 124 (1966); L. L. Le Shan, *You Can Fight for Your Life* (New York: M. Evans, 1977).

26. G. F. Solomon, "Emotions, Stress, the Central Nervous System and Immunity," *Annals of New York Academy of Sciences* 164 (1969), p. 6.

27. P. M. West, "Origin and Development of the Psychological Approach to the Cancer Problem," in *The Psychological Variables in Human Cancer* (Los Angeles: University of California Press, 1954), p. 19.

28. B. B. Brown, *New Mind, New Body* (New York: Bantam Books, 1975).

29. T. Everson and W. Cole, *Spontaneous Regression of Cancer* (Philadelphia: W. B. Saunders Co., 1966), p. 518; G. F. Solomon, "Emotions, Stress, the Central Nervous System and Immunity," *Annals of the New York Academy of Sciences* 164 (1969), p. 8.

30. Klopfer, "Psychological Variables;" Blumberg, "Psychological Factors and Cancer."

31. C. Binger, *The Doctor's Job* (New York: W. W. Norton, 1945).

32. A. Guggenbühl-Craig, *Power in the Healing Professions* (New York: Spring Publishers, 1971), p. 85; C. G. Jung, *Psyche and Symbol* (New York: Doubleday Anchor Books, 1958); C. G. Jung, *Four Archetypes* (Princeton, New Jersey: Princeton University Press, Bollingen Series, 1959).

33. Ibid.

34. O. C. Simonton and S. Simonton, "Belief Systems and Cancer," Seminar on Mind as Healer, Mind as Slayer, University of California, Berkeley, October 31, 1975.

35. Ibid.

Chapter 7: The Structure of Relationship

1. Kaplan et al., "Family Mediation of Stress."

2. Cantor, personal communications.

3. The majority of people with whom I have worked are white middle-class Americans. There is therefore an obvious cultural bias. This is especially true in the chapters on family patterns. And yet it seems to me that the fundamental experiences related to cancer come close to transcending cultural differences. The ideas and examples in this book come from the

white middle-class people with whom I have done most of my work, but I hope there is much here that is universal. And I trust further that appropriate modifications can be made by the reader when it is necessary to do so.

4. D. M. Kaplan, A. Smith, and R. Grobstein, "The Problems of Siblings," part of the proceedings of the American Cancer Society's National Conference on Human Values and Cancer, Atlanta, June 22, 1972, p. 140.

5. Cantor, personal communications.

6. D. J. Cantor, *Escape From Marriage* (New York: William Morrow, 1971).

7. These four patterns have been developed from the pioneering work of many investigators. I am particularly indebted to the following for their dynamic formulations: J. Barnett, "Narcissism and Dependency in the Obsessional-Hysteric Marriage," *Family Process* 11:4 (1972) for the concepts of "Obsessional-Narcissism" and "Hysterical Dependency"; Pincus, *Death and the Family* for the concepts of "Projection" and "Identification" Marriages; L. Wynne et al., "Pseudo-mutuality in the Family Relations of Schizophrenics," *Psychiatry* 21:205 (1958) for the concepts of "Pseudo-mutuality" and "Pseudo-hostility"; and most of all E. Shostrom and J. Kavanaugh, *Between Man and Woman* (New York: Bantam Books, 1975) for their concepts of "Nurturing, Supporting, Challenging, Educating, Comforting and Accommodating" relationship patterns.

8. V. Satir, *Peoplemaking* (Palo Alto: Science and Behavior Books, 1972), p. 137.

Chapter 8: The Hare-Tortoise Marriage Pattern

1. R. Cantor, personal communications.

2. Although the emotional tendencies associated with the Tortoise are usually experienced by the husband in our culture and those associated with the Hare usually by the wife, there are many instances in which the opposite is true: the husband experiences himself as emotional Hare, the wife as dependable Tortoise. For those interested in an excellent psychoanalytic discussion of this relationship pattern, see Barnett, "Narcissism and Dependency"; for a Jungian perspective on the same relationship tendencies, see E. Bertine, *Human Relationships* (New York: David McKay, 1958).

3. Henry James, *The Wings of the Dove* (New York: Dell, 1962), p. 53.

4. R. Cantor, personal communications.

5. Ibid.

6. Ibid.

7. Ibid.

8. Ibid.

9. Ibid.

10. Ibid.

11. Johnson, personal communications.

12. R. Cantor, personal communications.

13. Ibid.

14. Ibid.

15. Ms. Roach has written one of the most poignant and honest accounts of the cancer experience in existence. "The Last Day of April" was published by the American Cancer Society and is available through its state and local units.

Chapter 9: The Peacemaker Marriage Pattern

1. Margaret Mitchell, *Gone With the Wind* (New York: Macmillan, 1938).
2. The peacemaker pattern (also gladiator and parent-child) is based on the work of Shostrom and Kavanaugh (1975) and Wynne et al. (1958). I have expanded, illustrated and applied these concepts to the circumstances of the cancer crisis.
3. R. Cantor, personal communications.
4. Ibid.

Chapter 10: The Gladiator Marriage Pattern

1. Sutherland et al., *Psychological Impact of Cancer,* p. 85.
2. R. Cantor, personal communication between 1961 and 1977.
3. Ibid.
4. Ibid.
5. Ibid.
6. Ibid.
7. Ibid.

Chapter 11: The Parent-Child Marriage Pattern

1. R. Cantor, personal communications.
2. Ibid.
3. Ibid.
4. Ibid.

Chapter 12: Beyond Crime and Punishment

1. H. K. Beecher, "The Measurement of Pain," *Pharmacological Reviews* 9:190 (1957).
2. Victor E. Frankl, *Man's Search for Meaning* (New York: Pocket Books, 1971); and Victor E. Frankl, *The Doctor and the Soul* (New York: Vintage Books, 1973). Frankl has made meaning the core principle of his therapeutic work and writing. Many of the ideas developed in these chapters have their roots in his pioneering formulations.
3. Frankl, *Doctor and the Soul.*
4. Johnson, personal communications.

Chapter 13: God and Religious Belief

1. Johnson, personal communications between 1974 and 1977. Reverend Walter E. Johnson is a Presbyterian minister. He received his theological

training at the San Francisco Theological Seminary in San Anselmo, California and his psychotherapeutic training at the University of California Medical Center in San Francisco; Herrick Hospital in Berkeley, California; Duel Vocational Institute in Tracy, California; and the Family Therapy Center in San Francisco. He has been a hospital chaplain since 1964 and lives in Millbrae, California, with his wife, Esther, and their three children. Chapter Thirteen is based on our numerous conversations.

2. Ibid.
3. Genesis 18:24–32.
4. R. Cantor, personal communications.
5. Ibid.
6. Johnson, personal communications.

Chapter 14: Acts of Human Service

1. R. Cantor, personal communications.
2. Frankl, *Doctor and the Soul,* p. 56.
3. D. Renshaw, "How Patients and Their Families Cope with Cancer," *Medical Opinion* (August 1975), p. 22.
4. KCBS Radio interview with Nanette Fabray, August 29, 1975.
5. San Francisco *Chronicle,* October 17, 1976, p. 4.
6. Wilma King, Department of Genetics, Stanford Medical Center, Stanford, California.
7. T. Lasser, *Reach to Recovery* (New York: American Cancer Society, Inc., 1974), p. 11.
8. *Pacific Telephone Magazine* (January-February 1975), p. 13.
9. R. Cantor, personal communications.
10. Ibid.
11. Ibid.
12. Ibid.
13. Ibid.
14. Johnson, personal communications.
15. L. Horowitz, "Treatment of the Family with a Dying Member," *Family Process* 14:1 (1975), p. 59.
16. Johnson, personal communications.

Chapter 15: The Faith of Personal Experience

1. R. Cantor, personal communications.
2. Ibid.
3. Ibid.
4. Johnson, personal communications.
5. T. Wolfe, "The Me Decade," *New York* (August 23, 1976), p. 26.

References

Abrams, R. D. "The Patient with Cancer—His Changing Patterns of Communication, *New England Journal of Medicine,* 274:317, 1966.

———. "The Patient with Cancer," *Cancer,* 18:317, 1966a.

———. *Not Alone with Cancer.* Springfield, Ill.: C. C. Thomas, 1974.

———, and Finesinger, J. E. "Guilt Reactions in Cancer Patients," *Cancer,* 6:474, 1953.

Akehurst, A. C. "Post-Mastectomy Morale," *Lancet,* 2:181, 1972.

Ali, M. *The Greatest: My Own Story.* New York: Random House, 1975.

Alvarez, W. C. "Care of the Dying," *Journal of the American Medical Association,* 150:86, 1952.

Anderson, R. *After.* New York: Random House, 1974.

Annas, G. J. *The Rights of Hospital Patients.* New York: Avon Books, 1975.

Bahnson, C. B. "Psychophysiological Complementarity in Malignancies," *Annals of New York Academy of Sciences,* vol. 164, 1969.

Bakan, D. *Disease, Pain and Sacrifice.* Boston: Beacon Press, 1971.

Barckley, V. "Grief, A Part of Living," *Ohio's Health,* 20:34–38, 1968.

Bard, M., and Dyk, R. "The Psychodynamic Significance of Beliefs Regarding the Cause of Serious Illness," *Psychoanalytic Review,* 43:146, 1956.

Barnett, J. "Narcissism and Dependency in the Obsessional-Hysteric Marriage," *Family Process,* 11:4, 1972.

Becker, E. *The Denial of Death.* New York: The Free Press, 1973.

Beecher, H. K. "The Measurement of Pain," *Pharmacological Reviews,* 9:-190, 1957.

Bertine, E. *Human Relationships.* New York: David McKay, 1958.

Bibring, E. "The Mechanism of Depression," in Greenacre, P. (ed.), *Affective Disorders.* New York: International Universities Press, 1953.

Binger, C. *The Doctor's Job.* New York: W. W. Norton, 1945.

Blake, W. *Illustrations of the Book of Job* (introduction and interpretations by S. Foster Damon). New York: E. P. Dutton, 1969.

Blumberg, E. M., West, P. M., and Ellis, F. W. "A Possible Relationship Between Psychological Factors and Human Cancer," *Psychosomatic Medicine,* 16:4, 1954.

Boswell, J. *Life of Johnson.* Chapman, R. W., and Tinker, C. B. (ed.). New York: Oxford University Press, 1953.

Bouchard, R., and Owens, N. P. *Nursing Care of the Cancer Patient.* St. Louis: C. V. Mosby, 1972.

Bozeman, M. F., Orbach, C. E., and Sutherland, A. M. "Psychological Impact of Cancer—Its Treatment," *Cancer,* 8:1, 1955.

Branch, C. H. "Psychiatric Aspects of Malignant Disease," *Cancer,* 6:102, 1956.

Branden, N. *The Psychology of Self-Esteem.* New York: Bantam Books, 1973.

Brantner, J. "Life-Threatening Disease as a Manageable Crisis," *Seminars in Oncology,* 1:2, 1974.

Brown, B. B. *New Mind, New Body.* New York: Bantam Books, 1975.

Cameron, C. S. *The Truth about Cancer.* New York: Macmillan, 1967.

Cancer Facts and Figures. New York: American Cancer Society Publishers (214 E. 42nd St.), 1974.

Cantor, D. J. *Escape from Marriage.* New York: William Morrow, 1971.

Cantor, R. Personal communications with cancer patients and families and consultations with health professionals working with cancer patients and their families between 1961 and 1977.

———. "Orofacial Prosthetic Rehabilitation," *Archives of Otolaryngology,* vol. 87, 1968.

———. "Expression of Anger and Post-Surgical Adjustment," unpublished research completed at the University of California, San Francisco, 1970.

———. "Maxillofacial Rehabilitation," in Silverman, S., and Galante, M. *Oral Cancer.* San Francisco: University of California Press, 1966; second edition, 1972.

Caroline, N. S. "Dying in Academe," *The New Physician,* November, 1972.

Chernin, K. *Mothers and Daughters.* Unpublished manuscript used with permission of the author (1976).

Clayton, P. J. "The Effect of Living Alone on Bereavement Symptoms," *American Journal of Psychiatry,* 132:2, 1975.

Craig, T. J., and Abeloff, M. D. "Psychiatric Symptomatology Among Hospitalized Cancer Patients," *American Journal of Psychiatry,* 131:12, 1974.

Crammer, L. *Up from Depression.* New York: Pocket Books, 1972.

de Beauvoir, S. *A Very Easy Death.* New York: Warner Books, 1964.

Dovenmuehle, R. H., and Verwoerdt, A. "Physical Illness and Depressive Symptomatology," *Journal of Gerontology,* 18:260–266, 1963.

Easson, W. M. *The Dying Child.* Springfield, Ohio: C. C. Thomas, 1972.

Engel, G. L. *Psychological Development in Health and Disease.* Philadelphia: W. B. Saunders, 1962.

———. "A Life Setting Conducive to Illness: The Giving-Up/Given-Up Complex," *Annals of Internal Medicine,* 69:293–300, 1968.

Everson, T., and Cole, W. *Spontaneous Regression of Cancer.* Philadelphia: W. B. Saunders, 1966.

Feifel, H. (ed.). *The Meaning of Death.* New York: McGraw-Hill Book Co., 1959.

Fitts, W. T., and Raudin, I. S. "What Philadelphia Physicians Tell Patients with Cancer," *Journal of the American Medical Association,* 153:901, 1953.

Fixel, L. "Coming to This Place." Unpublished poem used by permission of the author.

Fogel, M. L., and Rosillo, R. H. "Correlation of Psychological Variables and Progress in Physical Rehabilitation," *Diseases of the Nervous System,* 30:9, 1969.

Francis, G. M. "Cancer: The Emotional Component," *American Journal of Nursing,* 69:8, 1969.

Frankl, V. E. *Man's Search for Meaning.* New York: Pocket Books, 1971.

_____. *The Doctor and the Soul.* New York: Vintage Books, 1973.

Freud, S. *Introductory Lectures in Psychoanalysis.* New York: Boni and Liveright, 1920.

_____. *Mourning and Melancholia,* in Collected Papers, IV. London: Hogarth Press, 1925.

_____. *The Problem of Anxiety.* New York: W. W. Norton, 1936.

Gallup Organization, Inc. "Women's Attitudes Regarding Breast Cancer," conducted for the American Cancer Society, 1974.

Garner, H. H. *Psychosomatic Management of the Patient with Malignancy.* Springfield, Ill.: C. C. Thomas, 1966.

Gerle, B., Lunden, G., and Sandblom, P. "The Patient with Inoperable Cancer from the Psychiatric and Social Standpoints," *Cancer,* 13:-1206, 1960.

Glasser, P., and Glasser, L. *Families in Crisis.* New York: Harper & Row, 1969.

Glick, I., Weiss, R., and Parkes, C. M. *The First Year of Bereavement.* New York: Wiley and Son, 1974.

Goffman, E. *Stigma.* Englewood Cliffs, N. J.: Prentice-Hall, 1963.

Gordon, D. C. *Overcoming the Fear of Death.* Baltimore: Penguin Books, 1972.

Graham, B. "Psychic and Cellular Aspects of Isolation and Identity Impairment in Cancer," *Annals of New York Academy of Sciences,* 164:352, 1969.

Grinker, R., and Spiegel, J. *Men Under Stress.* Philadelphia: Blakiston Co., 1945.

Guggenbühl-Craig, A. *Power in the Healing Professions.* New York: Spring Publishers, 1971.

Gunther, J. (interview with F. D. Adair). "Cancer in Our Breast," *Woman's Home Companion,* February 1954.

Hinkle, L. E., and Wolff, S. "A Summary of Experimental Evidence Relating Life Stress to Diabetes Mellitus," *Journal of Mt. Sinai Hospital,* 19:537–570, 1952.

Hinton, J. *Dying.* Baltimore: Penguin Books, 1967.

Holleb, A. I. "Cancer Therapy—The Patient's Choice?" *Cancer,* 33:301, 1974.

Horowitz, L. "Treatment of the Family with a Dying Member," *Family Process,* 14:1, 1975.

Hutschnecker, A. A. "Personality Factors in Dying Patients," in Feifel, H.

_____ (ed.), *The Meaning of Death*. New York: McGraw-Hill Book Co., 1953.

James, H. *The Wings of the Dove*. New York: Dell Publishing Co., 1962.

James, W. (ed.). *The Literary Remains of the Late Henry James*. Boston: Osgood Press, 1885.

_____. *The Principles of Psychology*. New York: Holt, Rinehart and Winston, 1890.

Johnson, W. E., Chaplain, Peninsula General Hospital, Millbrae, California. Personal communications between 1974 and 1977.

Jung, C. G. *Psyche and Symbol*. New York: Doubleday Anchor Books, 1958.

_____. *Four Archetypes*. Princeton, N. J.: Princeton University Press (Bollingen Series), 1959.

_____. (ed.). *Man and His Symbols*. Garden City, New York: Doubleday, 1968.

_____. *Two Essays on Analytical Psychology*. Cleveland: World Publishing Co., 1970.

Kaplan, D. M. "Observations on Crisis Theory and Practice," *Social Casework*, March 1968.

Kaplan, D. M., Smith, A., Grobstein, R., and Fischman, S. E. "Family Mediation of Stress," *Social Work*, July 1973.

Katz, J. L., Weiner, H., and Gallagher, T. F. "Stress, Distress and Ego Defenses," *Archives of General Psychiatry*, 23:131, 1970.

Klein, R. "A Crisis to Grow On," *Cancer*, December 1971.

Klopfer, B. "Psychological Variables in Human Cancer," *Journal of Projective Techniques*, 21:331, 1957.

Knapp, V. S., and Hansen, H. "Helping the Parents of Children with Leukemia," *Social Work*, July 1973.

Koenig, R. R. "Anticipating Death from Cancer—Physician and Patient Attitudes," *Michigan Medicine*, 68:17, 1969.

Kowal, S. J. "Emotions as a Cause of Cancer," *Psychoanalytic Review*, 42:3, 1955.

Kübler-Ross, E. *On Death and Dying*. New York: Macmillan, 1969.

_____. *Questions and Answers on Death and Dying*. New York: Collier Books, 1974.

Kushner, R. *Breast Cancer: A Personal History and an Investigative Report*. New York: Harcourt Brace Jovanovich, 1976.

Lasser, T. *Reach to Recovery*. New York: American Cancer Society, 1974.

LeShan, L. L. "Psychological States as Factors in the Development of Malignant Disease: A Critical Review," *Journal of the National Cancer Institute*, vol. 22, January 1959.

_____. "An Emotional Life-History Pattern Associated with Neoplastic Disease," *Annals of New York Academy of Sciences*, vol. 124, 1966.

_____. *You Can Fight for Your Life*. New York: M. Evans, 1977.

LeShan, L. L., and Worthington, R. E. "Personality as a Factor in the Pathogenesis of Cancer: A Review of the Literature," *British Journal of Medical Psychology*, vol. 29, 1956.

Lifton, R. J. "On Death and Death Symbolism: Horoshima Disaster," *Psychiatry*, 27:191, 1964.

Lindemann, E. "Symptomatology and Management of Acute Grief," *American Journal of Psychology*, 101:141, 1944.

Mannes, M. *Last Rights*. New York: Signet, 1975.

Miller, F. R., and Jones, H. W. "The Possibility of Precipitating the Leukemic State by Emotional Factors," *Blood*, 8:880, 1948.

Mitchell, M. *Gone With the Wind*. New York: Macmillan, 1938.

Montaigne, M. *Selected Essays*. New York: Pocket Books, 1959.

Moriarty, T. "A Nation of Willing Victims," *Psychology Today*, April 1975.

Murphy, L. B. *The Widening World of Childhood: Paths Toward Mastery*. New York: Basic Books, 1962.

Oken, D. "What to Tell Cancer Patients," *Journal of the American Medical Association*, 175:317, 1961.

Peck, A. "Emotional Reactions to Having Cancer," *Cancer*, 22:284, 1972.

Pelgrin, M. *And a Time to Die*. Sausalito: Contact Editions, 1962.

Pendergrass, E. P. "Host Resistance and Other Intangibles in the Treatment of Cancer," *American Journal of Roentgenology*, 85:891, 1961.

Pincus, L. *Death and the Family*. New York: Pantheon Books, 1974.

Quint, J. C. "The Impact of Mastectomy," *The American Journal of Nursing*, 63:11, 1963.

Renshaw, D. "How Patients and Their Families Cope with Cancer," *Medical Opinion*, August 1975.

Richards, V. *Cancer: The Wayward Cell*. Berkeley: University of California Press, 1972.

Robertson, D. *Survive the Savage Sea*. New York: Bantam Books, 1974.

Rosenthal, H. R. "Psychotherapy for the Dying," *American Journal of Psychotherapy*, 11:626, 1957.

Rothenberg, A. "Psychological Problems in Terminal Cancer Management," *Cancer*, 14:1063, 1961.

Rozen, R. D., Ordway, D., Curtis, T. A., and Cantor, R. "The Psycho-Social Aspects of Maxillofacial Rehabilitation: Part 1—The Effect of Primary Cancer Treatment," *Journal of Prosthetic Dentistry*, 28:4, 1972.

Satir, V. *Peoplemaking*. Palo Alto, California: Science and Behavior Books, 1972.

Schoenberg, B., Carr, A. C., Peretz, D., and Kutscher, A. H. (ed.). *Loss and Grief*. New York: Columbia University Press, 1970.

———. *Psychosocial Aspects of Terminal Care*. New York: Columbia University Press, 1972.

Schwartz, L. H., and Schwartz, J. L. *The Psychodynamics of Patient Care*. Englewood Cliffs, N. J.: Prentice-Hall, 1972.

Selye, H. *The Stress of Life*. New York: McGraw-Hill, 1966.

Shands, H. C., Finesinger, J. E., Cobb, S., and Abrams, R. D. "Psychological Mechanisms in Patients with Cancer," *Cancer*, 4:1159, 1951.

Shostrom, E., and Kavanaugh, J. *Between Man and Woman*. New York: Bantam Books, 1975.

Simonton, O. C., and Simonton, S. "Management of the Emotional Aspects of Malignancy," as part of a symposium *New Dimensions of Habilitation for the Handicapped,* Florida Department of Health and Rehabilitative Services, June 14, 1974.

_____. "Belief Systems and Cancer," Seminar on *Mind as Healer, Mind as Slayer,* University of California, Berkeley, October 31, 1975.

Solomon, G. F. "Emotions, Stress, the Central Nervous System and Immunity," *Annals of New York Academy of Sciences,* vol. 164, 1969.

Sutherland, A. M., et al. "Psychological Impact of Cancer and Cancer Surgery: Adaptation to the Dry Colostomy," *Cancer,* 5:5, 1952.

Sutherland, A. M., et al. *The Psychological Impact of Cancer.* New York: American Cancer Society, 1960.

Sutherland, A. M., and Bard, M. "Psychological Impact of Cancer and Its Treatment: Adaptation to Radical Mastectomy," *Cancer,* 8:4, 1955.

Sutherland, A. M., and Orback, C. E. "Psychological Impact of Cancer and Cancer Surgery: Depressive Reactions Associated with Surgery for Cancer," *Cancer,* 6:5, 1953.

Verwoerdt, A. "Communication with the Fatally Ill," *CA—A Cancer Journal for Clinicians,* 15:105–111, 1965.

Weisman, A. D. "The Patient with a Fatal Illness: To Tell or Not to Tell," *Journal of the American Medical Association,* 196:201, 1968.

_____. *On Dying and Denying.* New York: Behavioral Publications, 1973.

_____. *The Realization of Death.* New York: Jason Aronson, 1974.

West, P. M. "Origin and Development of the Psychological Approach to the Cancer Problem," in *The Psychological Variables in Human Cancer.* Los Angeles: University of California Press, 1954.

Wheelis, A. *How People Change.* New York: Harper & Row, 1973.

White, R. W. *The Abnormal Personality.* New York: Ronald Press, 1964.

_____. "Strategies of Adaptation: An Attempt at Systematic Description," in Coelho, G. V., Hamburg, D. A., and Adams, J. E. *Coping and Adaptation.* New York: Basic Books, 1974.

Wolfe, T. "The Me Decade," *New York,* August 23, 1976.

Wynne, L., Rychoff, I., Day, J., and Hirsch, S. "Pseudo-mutuality in the Family Relations of Schizophrenics," *Psychiatry,* 21:205–220, 1958.

Index